Frequently Asked Questions (FAQs)
for Postgraduate Practical Examination in
ORTHOPAEDICS

Frequently Asked Questions (FAQs)
for Postgraduate Practical Examination in
ORTHOPAEDICS
SECOND EDITION

KP Daga
MS (Orth) FCPS (Orth) D Orth Fellow of AO (Switzerland)

Formerly, Professor (Orthopaedics)
Padmashree Dr DY Patil Medical College, Mauritius
Examiner for MS (Orth)
Mauritius University
Head and Professor of Orthopaedics
Noble Medical College
Biratnagar, Nepal

Formerly, Professor of Orthopaedics
KBN Institute of Medical Sciences
Kalaburagi, Karnataka

Formerly, Associate Professor (Orthopaedics)
Dr VM Medical College
Solapur, Maharashtra, India

Foreword
L Prakash

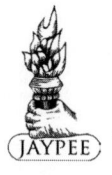

JAYPEE *The Health Sciences Publisher*
New Delhi | London | Panama

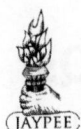 **Jaypee Brothers Medical Publishers (P) Ltd.**

Headquarters
Jaypee Brothers Medical Publishers (P) Ltd.
4838/24, Ansari Road, Daryaganj
New Delhi 110 002, India
Phone: +91-11-43574357
Fax: +91-11-43574314
E-mail: jaypee@jaypeebrothers.com

Overseas Offices

J.P. Medical Ltd.
83, Victoria Street, London
SW1H 0HW (UK)
Phone: +44 20 3170 8910
Fax: +44(0) 20 3008 6180
E-mail: info@jpmedpub.com

Jaypee Highlights Medical Publishers Inc.
City of Knowledge, Building 235, 2nd Floor
Clayton, Panama City, Panama
Phone: +1 507-301-0496
Fax: +1 507-301-0499
E-mail: cservice@jphmedical.com

Jaypee Brothers Medical Publishers (P) Ltd.
17/1-B, Babar Road, Block-B, Shaymali
Mohammadpur, Dhaka-1207
Bangladesh
Mobile: +08801912003485
E-mail: jaypeedhaka@gmail.com

Jaypee Brothers Medical Publishers (P) Ltd.
Bhotahity, Kathmandu, Nepal
Phone: +977-9741283608
E-mail: kathmandu@jaypeebrothers.com

Website: www.jaypeebrothers.com
Website: www.jaypeedigital.com

© 2018, Jaypee Brothers Medical Publishers

The views and opinions expressed in this book are solely those of the original contributor(s)/author(s) and do not necessarily represent those of editor(s) of the book.

All rights reserved. No part of this publication may be reproduced, stored or transmitted in any form or by any means, electronic, mechanical, photocopying, recording or otherwise, without the prior permission in writing of the publishers.

All brand names and product names used in this book are trade names, service marks, trademarks or registered trademarks of their respective owners. The publisher is not associated with any product or vendor mentioned in this book.

Medical knowledge and practice change constantly. This book is designed to provide accurate, authoritative information about the subject matter in question. However, readers are advised to check the most current information available on procedures included and check information from the manufacturer of each product to be administered, to verify the recommended dose, formula, method and duration of administration, adverse effects and contraindications. It is the responsibility of the practitioner to take all appropriate safety precautions. Neither the publisher nor the author(s)/editor(s) assume any liability for any injury and/or damage to persons or property arising from or related to use of material in this book.

This book is sold on the understanding that the publisher is not engaged in providing professional medical services. If such advice or services are required, the services of a competent medical professional should be sought.

Every effort has been made where necessary to contact holders of copyright to obtain permission to reproduce copyright material. If any have been inadvertently overlooked, the publisher will be pleased to make the necessary arrangements at the first opportunity. The **CD/DVD-ROM** (if any) provided in the sealed envelope with this book is complimentary and free of cost. **Not meant for sale.**

Inquiries for bulk sales may be solicited at: jaypee@jaypeebrothers.com

Frequently Asked Questions (FAQs) for Postgraduate Practical Examination in Orthopaedics

First Edition: 2006
Second Edition: **2018**

ISBN: 978-93-5270-361-6

Printed at Sanat Printers

Dedicated to

*My all postgraduate students of
past, present and future in orthopaedics*

Dr. L Prakash
M.B.B.S; M.S. (Orth); FASIF (Swiss); M.Ch. (Orth) (Liverpool); AOAA (Swiss)

Director & Chief of Orthopaedics

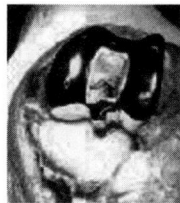

Institute for Special Orthopaedics (ISO 9001-2008 certified for Orthopaedic excellence)
29 Karuneegar street.
Nerkundram. Chennai 600107

Phone: +91 8144 311 311
www.prakash.tel
www.kneereplacement.in
www.drlprakash.com

Foreword

It is with great pleasure that I write this foreword to Dr KP Daga's *Frequently Asked Questions for Postgraduate Practical Examination in Orthopaedics*. In this twitter era, the young trainees and students seldom have time-to-read verbose texts or wade through voluminous material. However, most popular orthopaedic textbooks, written by native English speakers, has long complex sentences, and are taxing for the reader. In a significant departure from this trend, Dr Daga has written an extremely short and sweet book, which covers almost every aspect of orthopaedics.

Each short chapter takes up one topic, and each is described in the standard format of pointwise short sentences. The book will certainly become a must read for all orthopaedic undergraduates, early postgraduates, and those appearing for competitive examinations.

L Prakash

Preface to the Second Edition

Postgraduate examination can bring tension and terror to students. Due to this tension, many forget what they know at the time of examination and they cannot give proper answers and they are likely to fail even, if they know their subject well. To answer in practical examination is an art and needs presence of mind. One should have skill and methods of leading examiner to ask-desired questions, one can master this technique. This is called leading methods. But you should know the answer to these questions aroused via your examination.

Please tell your diagnosis first for being examined for short cases, then straight way tell your reasons for particular diagnosis. Then the discussion will lead to further part such as differential diagnosis, treatment. Please tell all standard methods of treatment in examinations and then go for latest and recent methods and discussion. You should reach to his part for your success. While making diagnosis, please tell common things first and do not tell rare diagnosis or syndromes. Please remember that if you examine more and more cases, it is beneficial for you.

Many chapters have been changed, altered and deleted as per developments in orthopaedics. I have tried to give some tips for postgraduate practical examinations in orthopaedics such as Diploma, MS and DNB. But this is not end. The sky is limit and there are endless questions and answers.

I have collected these questions through may experience of examinations as examinee, as examiner for many universities. I take this opportunity to thank all my colleagues, my friends, my teachers, co-examiners, for their help to collect and compile these questions and answers. I take this opportunity to thank, President-Principal, KBN Institute of Medical Sciences, Kalaburagi, Karnataka, India; Dean of Padmashree Dr DY Patil Medical College, Mauritius; and Drs Niranjan Kumar and Sunil Kumar Sharma, Nobel Medical College Teaching Hospital, Biratnagar, Nepal, for their help, cooperation, and suggestions.

I thank my wife, Ms KK Daga; my sons, Dr Ashutosh Daga, Mr Vaibhav Daga (Physiotherapist); my daughter, Mrs Sapna Kabra, my son-in-law; Mr Sandeep Kabra, my daughter-in-laws; and Mrs Manish Daga and Mrs Shilpi Daga, for their timely help and cooperation to complete this book.

I have been undergraduate and postgraduate examiner for various universities of India, and undergraduate and postgraduate teacher in orthopaedics of Shivaji University, Maharashtra, and Rajiv Gandhi University of Health Sciences (RGUHS), Karnataka, India.

Finally, I want to stress that the clinical examination with basic signs must be excellent, and then only you can progress, so please try to master basic clinical signs first.

KP Daga

Preface to the First Edition

Postgraduate examination can bring tension and terror to students. Due to this tension, many forget what they know at the time of examination and they cannot give proper answers and they are likely to fail even if they know their subject well. To answer in practical examination is an art and needs presence of mind. One should have skill and methods of leading examiner to ask-desired questions, one can master this technique. This is called leading methods. But you should know the answer to these questions aroused via your examination.

Be cool, do not loose temper, do not get nervous and answer to the point. If you do not know the answer please do not waste your time by keeping mum and let him ask next question and do not give up hopes, if you do not answer one or two questions. It is very important to answer many questions. Examiner wants to know what you know and what you have learnt and what you have studied and what you have retained and he is not interested to find out what you do not know.

Please tell your diagnosis first for being examined for short cases, then straight way tell your reasons for particular diagnosis. Then the discussion will lead to further part such as differential diagnosis, treatment. Please tell all standard methods of treatment in examinations and then go for latest and recent methods and discussion. You should reach to his part for your success. While making diagnosis, please tell common things first and do not tell rare diagnosis or syndromes. Please remember that if you examine more and more cases, it is beneficial for you.

I have tried to give some tips for Postgraduate Practical Examinations in Orthopaedics such as Diploma, MS and DNB. But this is not end. The sky is limit and there are endless questions and answers.

Try-to-face examination with these tips and success will be yours. I have collected these questions through may experience of examinations as examinee, as examiner for many universities. I take this opportunity to thank all my colleagues, my friends, my teachers, co-examiners, for their help to collect and compile these questions and answers.

I take this opportunity to thank the President, Principal, KBN Institute of Medical Sciences, Kalaburagi, for their help, cooperation and suggestions.

I thank my wife, Mrs KK Daga; my sons, Dr Ashutosh Daga, Mr Vaibhav Daga, (Physiotherapist); my daughter, Mrs Sapna Kabra; my son-in-law, Mr Sandeep Kabra; my daughter-in-laws, Mrs Manish Daga and Mrs Shilpi Daga, for their timely help and cooperation to complete this book.

I have been undergraduate and postgraduate examiner for many universities of India and undergraduate and postgraduate teacher in orthopaedics of Shivaji University Maharashtra, and Rajiv Gandhi University of Health Sciences (RGUHS) Karnataka, India.

Before concluding once again, I want to stress that the clinical examination with basic signs must be excellent, and then only you can progress, so please try to master basic clinical signs first.

KP Daga

Contents

1. Normal and Abnormal Gait — 1
2. Bone Infection (Osteomyelitis) — 4
3. Inflammatory Arthropathies — 9
4. Crystalline Arthropathies — 11
5. Rheumatoid Arthritis — 12
6. Osteoarthritis — 14
7. Septic Arthritis — 17
8. Diseases of Elbow — 21
9. Supracondylar Fracture of Humerus and Cubitus Varus — 25
10. Elbow Dislocations and Instability — 29
11. Nerve Entrapments of Elbow, Forearm, Wrist and Hand — 31
12. Claw Hand due to Hansen's Disease — 35
13. Congenital Disorders — 40
14. Clubfoot — 50
15. Foot Drop — 55
16. Evaluation of Hip Disease — 56
17. Tubercular Infection of Hip Joint — 63
18. Slipped Capital Femoral Epiphysis — 67
19. Legg-Calvé-Perthes Disease — 69
20. Fracture Neck of Femur — 72
21. Intertrochanteric Fracture — 79
22. Total Hip Replacement — 82

23. Recurrent Dislocation of Patella — 88
24. Evaluation of Knee Joint — 90
25. Total Knee Arthroplasty — 96
26. Problems of Spine — 102
27. Tuberculous Infection of Spine — 111
28. Poliomyelitis — 116
29. Volkmann's Ischemic Contracture — 120
30. Non-union — 122
31. Different Methods of Fracture Fixation — 127
32. Ilizarov Technique — 132
33. Metabolic and Endocrine Disorders — 134
34. The Art of Physiotherapy — 136
35. Orthoses, Braces, Splints — 138
36. Protheses — 147
37. Diagnostic Radiology — 148
38. Computed Tomography and Magnetic Resonance Imaging — 154
39. Nuclear Medicine — 159
40. Ward Rounds, Suture Materials, Methods of Sterilisation and OT Techniques — 161
41. Miscellaneous Affections — 167
42. Commonly Accepted Classifications in Orthopaedics — 183
43. International and National Orthopaedic Surgeons Who Have Contributed to World of Orthopaedics — 200

Bibliography — *207*

CHAPTER 1

Normal and Abnormal Gait

Q.1 What are the phases of normal gait?
Ans. There are two phases of normal gait:
1. *Stance phase (60% of the gait cycle):* When the foot is on the ground (heel strike), foot flat, midstance, and push off (toe off).
2. *Swing phase (40% of the gait cycle):* When foot is moving forward—acceleration, midswing and deceleration.

Q.2 What is width of normal base?
Ans. It is usually 2–4 inches.

Q.3 What is normal step length?
Ans. It is approximately 15 inches.

Q.4 How much pelvis and trunk shifting normally?
Ans. Pelvis and trunk shifts laterally approximately 1 inch during gait to weight-bearing side to center weight over the hip.

Q.5 How much pelvis rotates during normal gait?
Ans. During swing phase, pelvis rotates 40° forward while opposite hip acts as fulcrum.

Q.6 How many steps one can walk in one minute normally?
Ans. One can walk 90–120 steps per minute, which is called cadence.

Q.7 What are different types of pathological gait?
Ans. They are:
- Trendelenburg gait
- Antalgic gait
- Waddling gait
- Short-leg gait
- Stiff-hip gait
- Stiff-knee gait
- Scissors gait
- Spastic gait
- Propulsive gait

These gaits are found in neurological conditions (polio):
- Flat-foot gait
- Hand-to-knee gait
- High-step gait
- Calcaneal gait.

Q.8 What is Trendelenburg gait?

Ans. This is due to weakness of gluteus medius muscle which may be seen in coax vara, fractures of greater trochanter, polio, lesion of nerve of the muscle. Here weak gluteus medius muscle acts as tie-rod since it prevents unsupported hip from dropping down and causing instability and the patient exhibits typical abduction lurch.

Q.9 What is antalgic gait?

Ans. When there is pain, the patient tries to avoid to put weight on one leg and takes off weight as early as possible during stance phase. This may be seen in hip diseases and shoe problems.

Q.10 What is waddling gait?

Ans. When the patient has weak abduction mechanism on both sides and there is bilateral Trendelenburg lurch, the patient walks with moving both sides (lurching) commonly seen in bilateral dysplasia of the hip (CDH).

Q.11 What is hand-to-knee gait?

Ans. During stance phase, the knee is in extension in normal gait but when there is weak quadriceps or fusion of knee, the patient cannot do extension and for that, the patient has to push limb with the hand. This is also called unstable knee gait.

Q.12 What is high-step gait?

Ans. This is seen in foot drop seen after affection of lateral popliteal nerve, may be after Hansen's disease, and traumatic peroneal nerve affection. Due to weakness of dorsiflexors, there is slapping down of foot after heel strike.

Q.13 What is gait in painful heel?

Ans. When there is painful calcaneal spur or spike, then the patient tries to avoid heel strike completely and hops onto the involved foot.

Q.14 What are different types of lurching gaits?

Ans.
- Weakness of gluteus medius—abduction lurching type
- Weakness of gluteus maximus—extension lurching type.

Q.15 What is difference between lurch and limp?

Ans.
- Limp—any deformity gait
- Lurch—swaying off of pelvis or trunk to avoid weight.

Q.16 How do you describe gait of abduction deformity with stiff hip?
Ans. Patient sways to opposite side to clear off the ground.

Q.17 What are major movements during gait?
Ans.
- Propulsion with plantar flexion of foot and toes
- Extension of hip joint followed by abduction and external rotation for next phase extension of knee joint.

Q.18 What is load on full-weight bearing through the hip joint?
Ans.
- Usually 350 lbs per sq inch
- When one stands on one limb, 3 times weight passes through other weight-bearing limb.

Q.19 What is calcaneal gait?
Ans. When gastrocnemius, soleus, and flexor hallucis logus are weak, lead to flat footed or calcaneal gait as these muscles are vital for push off.

Q.20 What is back-knee gait?
Ans. When hamstrings are weak, heel strike in deceleration may be excessively harsh, causing thickening of heel pad and knee gets hyperextended or back-knee gait.

Q.21 What is ataxic gait?
Ans. Ataxic or broad-based gait is due to—acute cerebellar ataxia, alcohol intoxication, brain injury, damage to nerve cells in the cerebellum of the brain (cerebellar degeneration), medications (phenytoin and other seizure medications), polyneuropathy (damage to many nerves, as occurs with diabetes).

CHAPTER 2

Bone Infection (Osteomyelitis)

Q.1 What is osteomyelitis?
Ans. It is the infection of all layers of bone.

Q.2 What are types of osteomyelitis?
Ans. *Acute osteomyelitis:* Hematogenous systemic illness of less than 10 days without history of previous episode.
Subacute osteomyelitis: No systemic symptoms, with radiological changes, duration more than 10 days.
Chronic osteomyelitis: Duration more than one month, history of previous episode, radiological bony changes with or without systemic illness.

Q.3 What is acute osteomyelitis?
Ans. This is an acute infection of medullary canal with increased osteolytic activity, fat necrosis. Pathogens are passed through least resistant part causing periosteal abscess, ultimate result depends upon virulence of organism, resistance of host and local conditions.

Q.4 How do you diagnose an acute osteomyelitis clinically?
Ans. Severe localized bony pain and tenderness, soft tissue inflammation, fever (variable), loss of function of adjacent joint 12–48 hours after onset, painful and tense joint effusion either of septic arthritis or sterile effusion.

Q.5 What pathological tests are done to diagnose osteomyelitis?
Ans.
- ESR—highly raised (more of prognostic value)
- C-reactive protein—raised
- Blood culture—75% cases, this is positive and guile for organism, within 48–72 hours.
- Aspiration of fluid or pus of abscess also gives idea about organisms either by microscopic or culture examination.

Q.6 Why area of metaphysis is commonly involved?
Ans. Vessels at metaphysic have hair pin bend, tortuous course, sluggish blood flow, nidus for bacteria, rapidly growing end and due to trauma and weight bearing (physiological loading), there may be microfracture and thus due to increased blood supply, the area of metaphysis is commonly affected.

Q.7 What are radiological ways to diagnose osteomyelitis?

Ans. Plain X-ray shows changes after at least 10 days after onset of disease, such as periosteal reaction, thickening, lytic lesions can be seen between 2-6 weeks after onset of disease, sclerotic changes are seen in chronic osteomyelitis. Soft tissue oedema of surrounding tissue may be present in 35-50% cases.

Radiolnuclide scanning—more sensitive than plain X-ray. Changes can be seen quite early.

Magnetic resonance imaging—quite sensitive even within 24-72 hours of onset of disease, helpful in diagnosing, extent of disease, better anatomic details, localisation can also be done specifically, and helps in localising aspiration of pus or site of biopsy, can detect early marrow oedema, periosteal reaction, sequestrum formation.

Computed tomography (CT)—good for differentiation between bone and soft tissue infections, but not as useful as MRI.

Q.8 At what stage are radiological changes seen on plain X-ray in osteomyelitis?

Ans. When changes are seen on plain X-ray, the disease is either subacute or chronic. It takes few days:
- Subacute—usually lytic lesion is seen
- Chronic—sequestrum and involucrum are present.

Q.9 What is picture of untreated osteomyelitis?

Ans. Local abscess, bony absorption in patches, periostitis, periosteal abscess.

Q.10 What is sequestrum?

Ans. It is dead piece of bone lying in pool of pus.

Q.11 What is involucrum?

Ans. This is new cortical bone laid down by periosteum around old bone (sequestrum).

Q.12 What are types of sequestrum?

Ans. Flake sequestrum, tubular sequestrum, ring sequestrum, coral form sequestrum, colored sequestrum, ivory sequestrum, coarse sand-like sequestrum, feathery sequestrum, Bombay nigra sequestrum, muscle sequestrum.

Q.13 What are common organisms in osteomyelitis?

Ans. Mainly they are *Staphylococcus aureus*, less commonly, *Streptococcus* Gram-negative bacilli.

Q.14 What is Cierny and Mader (1981) classification of chronic osteomyelitis?

Ans.
- *Anatomic Type I:* It medullary osteomyelitis–hematogenous and infected fracture non-union. This is primarily endosteal disease, may be sequelae of medullary fixation-infected

- *Type II:* Superficial osteomyelitis
- *Type III:* localized infection with sequestrum, cavitation
- *Type IV:* Diffuse osteomyelitis—combination of Type I, II, III and with instability.

Q.15 What is Brodie's abscess?
Ans. This is form of chronic osteomyelitis. This is encapsulated abscess in the bone surrounded by sclerotic margin with or without sequestrum in the cavity which is filled with pus or fluid which may be sterile. There is osteolytic lesion. Clinically, patient complains of dull aching pain at the site of lesion.

Q.16 What is treatment of Brodie's abscess?
Ans. Decompression with excision of lesion with sclerotic margin till one gets normal bone margin with or without continuous saline irrigation for few days with either saline or selected antibiotics as per culture report.

Q.17 Where do you get bilateral osteomyelitis?
Ans. When there is *Salmonella* osteomyelitis in cases of sickle cell anemia.

Q.18 How do you define sclerosing osteomyelitis of Garre?
Ans. This is subacute form of osteomyelitis, with lowgrade infection with patchy sclerosis in long bones at diaphysis.

Q.19 What is the treatment of chronic osteomyelitis?
Ans. This is staged as follows—*First stage:* Adequate debridement and curettage with or without antibiotic-laden cement depots in the form of beads or dowels. *Second stage* is of placement of bone grafts and fixation of bone if needed.

Saucerisation with or without filling cavity by bone grafts or muscle flaps principle is that by making shallow cavity so as there should not be any collection.

Closed suction irrigation (Carel and Dakin's method)—with or without gentamicin or tobramycin beads. Which may be removed after 10–14 days after formation of granulation, tissue otherwise it is difficult to remove them.

Intramedullary reaming is good way of debridement for diaphyseal involvement.

Q.20 What is Bier's method?
Ans. Putting Maggots and liquid paraffin in the wound to get sealed cavity by scavenging.

Q.21 What is Halstead's method?
Ans. This is electromagnetic induction of chronic infection which started in 1984.

Q.22 How cavities after osteomyelitis are closed after operation?
Ans. By bone grafts, muscle flaps and gentamicin or tobramycin beads.

Q.23 What is Papineau Rhinelanders' method?
Ans. This is divided in four stages:
1. Debridement
2. Saucerisation
3. Bone grafts with or without myocutaneous flaps
4. External fixators for stability.

Q.24 What are common complications after chronic osteomyelitis?
Ans.
- Shortening or lengthening (5% cases)
- Pathological fractures
- Septic arthritis
- Joint stiffness
- Contracture of joints especially flexion contracture
- Secondary skin infection
- Amyloidosis
- Generalised septicemia or bacteraemia
- Squamous cell carcinoma at sinus.

Q.25 What are the causes of death in osteomyelitis?
Ans. Without proper treatment, the patients may die of thromboembolism, amyloidosis and sqamous cell carcinoma.

Q.26 How do you diagnose chronic osteomyelitis on X-ray?
Ans. By presence of sequestrum as seen as sclerosed piece of bone in the cavity with involucrum, bony irregularity (due to periosteal reaction) and improper remodeling after healing of sinuses and cavities.

Q.27 Where do you use methylene blue?
Ans. This is used at the time of operation of sinus excision. When injected through sinus it demarcates the dead tissue by staining blue by living tissue stained as grey.

Q.28 How do you differentiate sequestrum from living bone?
Ans. Sequestrum may be ivory, pale white, rough surface on one side, smooth on other side, lies in pus, seen sclerosed piece on X-ray. Heavy sinks in water.
Living bone-bleeds on removal, floats in water.

Q.29 What are success rate of treatment of osteomyelitis?
Ans.
- *Type I*—If treated as per protocol such as debridement by intramedullary reaming or saucerisation, closure of dead space by antibiotic-laden cement, bone grafting or muscle flap, etc. success rate is 89% to 100%.
- *Type II*—When treated by drainage and curettage—success rate is 79% to 100%

- *Type III*—By simple stabilisation and closure of dead space, combination of methods used for type I and type II are used with or without antibiotic-laden cement, followed by reconstruction. Success rate is 92 to 98%.
- *Type IV*—Complex stabilisation, dead space closure, reconstruction after removal of dead bones, gap is filled, leads to 80 to 98% success.

Q.30 Summarise the picture of osteomyelitis as per age and clinical behavior and treatment.

Ans.

	Infancy	*Childhood*	*Adult*
1.	Secondary to umbilical inf.	Hematogenous	Open fracture
2.	Less constitutional symptoms	More	Moderate
3	*Site:* Intraarticular Metaphyseal and epiphyseal	Metaphyseal	Diaphyseal
4.	Local temperature—raised little	Raised	Moderately raised
5.	Periosteum perforated by pus	Subperiosteal abscess adherent	Periosteum
6.	Frequent joint affection as vessels passing through epiphysis and growth plate	Less frequent muscular adhesions	In late cases due to
7.	Less sequestrum	Very common	Smaller thin
8.	Shortening	Shortening or lengthening	No effect

CHAPTER 3

Inflammatory Arthropathies

Q.1 What are seronegative spondyloarthropathies?
Ans. The seronegative spondyloarthropathies are a group of rheumatic disease sharing common clinical, genetic and radiological features, such as ankylosing spondylitis, Reiter's syndrome, arthropathies with bowel diseases.

Q.2 What are common features of seronegative spondyloarthropathies?
Ans.
- Usually axial skeleton is affected by inflammatory lesions
- Oligoarticular peripheral joint arthritis
- Inflammation at bony insertions of tendons, ligaments and articular capsules
- Associated frequently with extra-articular inflammation of eye (uveitis), heart (aortitis), skin and mucosal membranes
- Usually young adults are affected
- Strong association with HLA-B27
- Negative rheumatic factor.

Q.3 What are ways to diagnose ankylosing spondylitis?
Ans. By clinical feature, onset before 40 years, insidious onset, daily symptoms for more than 3 months, prolonged morning stiffness, and improvement of symptoms by exercises other ways. X-ray first to show involvement of sacroiliac joint (absolutely essential) shows (AP views) bilateral SI arthritis, can be helped by CT scan with compatible history and physical examination with extra-skeletal involvement such as acute uveitis.

Q.4 What are treatment modalities for ankylosing spondylitis (AS)?
Ans.
- Nonsteroidal anti-inflammatory drugs
- ESP indomethacin
- Education of patient
- Physical therapy—back extension exercises, exercises for improvement of range of motions can be taught and done at home.

Q.5 What is disability in AS?

Ans. Affected patient less than 20% have significant disability there is usually deterioration of movements of hip leading to fusion of hip and spine (bamboo spine).

Q.6 What is reactive arthritis?

Ans. Reactive arthritis is joint inflammation initiated by an infection in which causative agent cannot be isolated from the joint. Reactive arthritis is included in the family of spondyloarthropathies.

Q.7 What is symptom complex of classic reactive arthritis [Reiter's syndrome]?

Ans. Usually GI tract infection and urogenital tract infections are precipitating factors.

The symptom complex includes: Infection of GI tract or genitals, these are barely symptomatic urethritis, conjunctivitis, cervicitis, mucocutaneous lesions—which are keratoderma, balanitis of penis, oral ulceration and changes in nail and arthritis or spondylitis. Musculoskeletal manifestations which are oligoarthritis, dactylitis, spondylolitis, sacroiliitis, but these develop 1-4 weeks after infection.

Reactive arthritis with musculoskeletal system and without other manifestations is called incomplete Reiter's syndrome, which occurs in approximately 40% of patients.

CHAPTER 4

Crystalline Arthropathies

Q.1 What are major clinical crystalline arthropathies?
Ans.
- Monosodium urate arthropathy
- Calcium pyrophosphate deposition disease (CPPD).

Q.2 How many types of gouty arthropathies?
Ans.
- Acute inflammatory arthritis
- Chronic erosive tophaceous arthritis.

Q.3 What are joints commonly involved in gout arthritis?
Ans. Usually the attack is of metatarsophalangeal joint of great toe. Other joints which are involved are as follows—ankles, knees, wrists, fingers, and elbows. Distal and joints of lower extremity are commonly involved.

Q.4 What are laboratory test help in diagnosis of acute gout or acute pseudogout?
Ans.
- Joint aspiration and analysis of aspirated fluid such as cell count, crystalline analysis under polarized microscope for appropriate crystals such as monosodium in acute gout and calcium pyrophosphate in acute pseudogout.
- Gram stain and routine culture and sensitivity.
- Routine X-rays are usually normal finding chondrocalcinosis on plain X-ray leads to clue of acute pseudogout.

CHAPTER 5

Rheumatoid Arthritis

Q.1 What is the definition of rheumatoid arthritis?
Ans. Rheumatoid arthritis (RA) is symmetric inflammatory arthritis involving small joints and large joints at least for 6 weeks.

Q.2 What is pattern of onset of RA?
Ans. Usually, the onset is insidious, slow and for weeks to months. With accompanied symptoms such as fatigue, malaise, anorexia, loss of weight, myalgia, arthralgia, morning stiffness, some may have acute or subacute onset also.

Q.3 What are diagnostic criteria for RA?
Ans.
- Morning stiffness.
- Arthritis for at least 3 weeks and lasting for more than 6 weeks.
- Arthritis of hand joints lasting for more than 6 weeks.
- Symmetric arthritis lasting more than 6 weeks.
- Radiologic changes.
- Serum rheumatoid factor.
- Rheumatoid arthritis.

Q.4 What are joints commonly involved?
Ans. They are wrist, metacarpophalangeal and proximal interphalangeal joints, knees, ankles and metatarsophalangeal joints, shoulders, hips, elbows.

Q.5 What are common drugs used for RA?
Ans. Narcotic analgesics, corticosteroids, nonsteroidal anti-inflammatory drugs (NSAIDs) and disease-modifying agents such as plaquenil, methotrexate and parental gold.

Q.6 What are extra-articular lesions of RA?
Ans. They are nodules, dry eyes, dry mouth, and carpal tunnel syndrome.

Q.7 What is the role of steroids in RA?
Ans. Many patients show good improvement with conservative use of corticosteroids. Males are given does of 7.5 mg of prednisone and females are

given 5 mg in morning. This system is followed for long term without any adverse effects and well tolerated sometimes selective long acting injections in the joints may be very effective.

Q.8. What is indication of disease-modifying treatment for RA?

Ans. Patients who do not respond to usual treatment of steroid and NSAID need additional method of treatment of disease-modifying agents are plaquenil, methotrexate and parental gold.

Q.9 What is role of synovectomy in RA?

Ans. Synovectomy is done to relieve pain of RA. The major indication of synovectomy at present is extensor synovectomy for prophylaxis of rupture of extensor tendons.

CHAPTER 6

Osteoarthritis

Q.1 What is osteoarthritis?

Ans. Osteoarthritis (OA) is noninflammatory disorder of joint where there is deterioration of articular cartilage and formation of new bone at joint and margins of bone called osteophytes. This is also known as degenerative joint disease.

Q.2 What are important causative factors of OA?

Ans. Obesity, genetics and heredity, particular occupation, multiple endocrine disorders, multiple metabolic disorders.

Q.3 What are pathological findings of OA?

Ans. Early degeneration of articular cartilage surface in the form of flaking or fibrillation in the weight-bearing joints, leading to complete loss of articular cartilage and eburnation of bone which is highly polished with sclerotic surface, cysts may occur in subchondral bone usually at weight-bearing areas may be due to microfractures which degenerate, formation of new bone at base of articular cartilage and surrounding the cyst creating an area of sclerosis.

Q.4 What are osteophytes? Why do they form?

Ans. These are marginal of ossified cartilage outgrowths. Due to vascularization in the subchondral bone, proliferation of adjacent cartilage and endochondral ossification occur and these extend from free articular space along with path of least resistance and try to increase the weight-bearing surface.

Q.5 How do you correlate pathologic abnormalities with radiological findings?

Ans.
- Cartilage erosion—loss of joint space
- Increased cellularity and deposition of bone at subchondral area—bone eburnation
- Intrusion of synovial fluid into bone-subchondral cysts
- Revascularisation of remaining cartilage and capsular traction—formation of osteophytes
- Synovial membrane stimulation—formation of osteophytes
- Compression of weakened bone—collapse of bone
- Fragmentation of osteochondral surface—formation of loose bodies.
- Destruction and distortion of capsular ligaments-deformities and malalignment.

Q.6 What is symptomatology of OA?

Ans. Main symptoms are pain during movements of joint and relieved by rest, which is aching in character and without localization. In advanced stage, the pain is there even at rest, sleep is disturbed by pain, movements are painful and restricted, muscle spasm, morning stiffness, pain after long rest, crepitations, sometimes contractures causing deformity such as flexion.

Q.7 What are clinical signs of OA?

Ans. Localized tenderness more along area of degeneration, palpable osteophytes, crepitations during range of movements, minimal effusion, which may be more after trivial trauma.

Aspirated synovial fluid is noninflammatory, with good viscosity without any other abnormality.

Q.8 What are radiological abnormalities?

Ans. Scanning with 99m-technetium shows increased uptake around OA joints, MRI reveal degenerative changes, subchondral cysts, osteophytes. CT scan also shows same things.

Q.9 What are complications of OA?

Ans.
- With loss of joint space angulation may occur creating deformity of the joint, such as knee
- Subluxation may occur such as carpometacarpal joint of thumb
- Ankylosis or complete bony fusion may occur such as in great toe
- Formation of loose bodies may be after subchondral microfractures.

Q.10 What are diseases which lead to secondary OA?

Ans. Acute and chronic trauma, Wilson's disease, acromegaly, alcaptonuria, hemophilia, syringomyelia, hyperparathyroidism, frostbite, overuse of steroids, neurologic disorders.

Q.11 What is Heberden's node?

Ans. Heberden's nodes are palpable bony enlargements about distal interphalangeal joints of hands.

Q.12 What is Bouchard's node?

Ans. Bouchard's nodes are bony enlargements of proximal interphalangeal joints.

Q.13 What is mucinous cyst?

Ans. Mucinous cysts arise from joint capsule in the distal or proximal interphalangeal joints, usually they contain degenerative myxomatous fibrous tissue arisen from degenerative arthritis.

Q.14. What are causes of degenerative arthritis of wrist?

Ans.
- Trauma
- Nonunion of scaphoid

- Gout
- CCPD disease
- Kienbock's disease—osteonecrosis of lunette
- Carpal instability by disruption of ligaments.

Q.15 What is bunion?
Ans. Bunion is combination of degenerative disease with angulation (valgus) of first metatarsal phalangeal joint with symptoms of progressive swelling and pain with difficulty in wearing of shoes and walking, inflammation of bursa on medial aspect of joint.

Q.16 What are finding with OA of hip?
Ans. Reduction of joint space which is seen on anteroposterior X-ray of hip with osteophytes, at inferior or superior border of acetabulum, superior or inferior to femoral head, loose bodies may be seen, sclerosis of underlying bone with adjacent bony cysts which may be in head, neck and acetabular area, painful and some restriction of movements.

Q.17 What is erosive osteoarthritis?
Ans. Erosive osteoarthritis involves primarily distal and proximal interphalangeal joints, which may be hereditary with severe inflammatory episodes leading to deformities and ankylosis, cysts may be tender and painful with frequent affection of post-menopausal women, with severe destruction of joint, X-ray shows severe bony erosion with sclerosis.

Q.18 What are new methods of treatment for OA and cartilage defects?
Ans.
- *Soft tissue grafts:* Periosteal or perichondral grafts are sewn over cartilage defects such as small piece of rib perichondrium transplanted.
- *Chondrocyte transplantation:* Articular cartilage is harvested by arthroscope and chondrocytes are cultured and grown in the laboratory and then placed over defects. Periosteal flap is sutured over that medial chondylar defects of femur are being treated with encouraging results.
- *Mosaic grafts:* Mosaic grafts are autogratfs. Osteochondral plugs are taken from peripheral areas of anteromedial or anterolateral femoral condyles. Corresponding holes are drilled to match size and depth of plug in the chondral defects which are then inserted into the defects which create look of mosaic look.
- *Artificial matrix:* Caron fibers, collagen, bone matrix, and polylactic acid are being tried to fill defects upon which cartilage can grow.
- Fresh osteochondral grafts are also being tried.
- Techniques include lavage and debridement, abrasion arthroplasty, subchondral penetration procedures (drilling and microfracture), and laser/thermal chondroplasty.

Q.19 What is role of stem cell therapy in OA?
Ans. Stem cells regenerate the degenerated cells and cause repair of tissue and get relief of symptoms.

CHAPTER 7

Septic Arthritis

Q.1 What is septic arthritis?
Ans. Septic arthritis is bacterial infection of the symposium and joint space causing profuse inflammatory reaction with migration of polymorphs leukocytes and release of proteolytic enzymes causing fast destruction of the joint and one third of patients have residual loss of function.

Q.2 What is process of articular damage in septic arthritis?
Ans. Bacteria in the synovium gets multiplied and release products from bacteria, which stimulate migration of polymorphs leukocytes into the joint, which release proteolytic enzymes which in turn cause acute and mild to severe damage to articular cartilage.

Q.3 What are predisposing conditions for septic arthritis?
Ans. These are trauma, diabetes mellitus, renal failure, malignancy, vascular insufficiency, recent joint infection, rheumatoid arthritis, steroid administration, immunosuppressive drug abuse, etc.

Q.4 What are common site which are affected with septic arthritis?
Ans. They are knee: 53%, hip: 20%, shoulder: 11%, elbow: 17%, wrist: 9% and ankle: 8%.

Q.5 What are clinical classification of septic arthritis?
Ans. They are:
- Acute monoarticular septic arthritis
- Chronic monoarticular septic arthritis
- Polyarticular septic arthritis

Q.6 What are tests for diagnosis of septic arthritis?
Ans. They are:
- Complete blood count with differential count
- Erythrocyte sedimentation rate (prognostic value)
- C-reactive protein
- Blood culture
- Plain X-rays
- Examination of aspirated fluid either transudate or exudates (this is most accurate diagnostic tool for diagnosis)

Q.7 What are diagnostic tests for aspirated fluid of septic arthritis?
Ans.
- Gram stain—positive gram stain is found in 60% cases, Gram-+ve cocci culture and sensitivity
- Glucose level is low
- Crystals—usually negative for uric acid and calcium pyrophosphate
- WBC count (total and differential) is increased, may be more than 50000 per square mm, polymorphs is 80%.

Q.8 What is clinical picture of septic arthritis?
Ans. Clinical picture depends upon age and self-defensive mechanism of an individual.
- Acute septic arthritis in older children and adults, presents—acute onset in terms of hours to few days, pain, swelling, limitation of movements of joint, fever (50–70% cases)
- In neonates, immune system is not fully mature so typical inflammatory response as in older children is not present, may be mild swelling, tenderness, irritability, discomfort of joint movements, and pseudoparalysis of the affected limb.

Q.9 What is clinical presentation and microbiology of chronic monoarticular septic arthritis?
Ans.
- It depends upon the duration when patient is presented.
- Early stage—low-grade synovitis pain swelling, warmth, and erythema. This occurs in patients with low immune system such as patients with rheumatoid arthritis, lupus erythematous, chronic dialysis, renal transplant.
- The common organisms which are found are—mycobacteria, fungi, saprophytic bacteria; which get introduced into the joint either by hematogenous spread, spread along planes of low resistance, or directly by penetrating trauma, surgery, or arthrocentesis and lead-top tissue destruction by mononuclear cell and giant cell infiltration.
- Late stage—all signs and symptoms of chronic infection, with extensive tissue destruction with radiological changes.

Q.10 What is clinical picture of polyarticular septic arthritis?
Ans. Polyarticular septic arthritis (PASA) occurs in 5–8% of children and 10–19% in nongonococcal in adult cases.

In gonococcal arthritis, majority of patients present with multiple joint pains, and patients are usually are young, healthy, sexually active and only 20–50% cases give positive culture report. There are many predisposing conditions such as rheumatoid arthritis, diabetes, over use of corticosteroid drugs, renal failure, parental drug abuse where multiple joints are involved and the patients are elderly and chronically ill with mortality rate of 25–50%. The most common organism isolated is *S. aureus* and sometimes *Neisseria spp, Streptococcus, Pneumococcus,* and *H. influenzae.*

Septic Arthritis

Q.11 What are common organisms found in septic arthritis of neonates children, young adults, and elderly people?

Ans.
- In neonates, *S. aureus*, B. streptococci, Gram negative *N. gonorrhoeae*
- In children (2 months to 2 years) *H. influenzae*, *S. aureus*, streptococci, and *H. influenzae*
- In young adults, *S. aureus*, *N. gonorrhoeae*—most common, 25% cases
- In elderly—*S. aureus*, 45-64% cases Gram negative bacilli are seen in 14-35% cases.

Q.12 What is clinical picture of gonococcal arthritis?

Ans. Disseminated gonococcal infection (DGI) is term given to describe *N. gonorrhoeae* bacteremia and 0.5-3% individuals develop clinical manifestations of DGI and out of that 17-33% patients develop septic arthritis. Starting symptoms of DGI are migratory or additive multiple joint pains (70%), tenosynovitis (67%), dermatitis (67%), fever (63%), and arthritis (42%). Tenosynovitis is common to multiple joints but especially wrists, fingers, ankles, and toes. The dermatitis consists of multiple painless skin lesions usually found on extremities and trunk, may in the form of haemorrhagic maculas or papules some times pustules, vesicles and bullae genitourinary symptoms are usually absent.

There are two types of clinical presentations of arthritis in DGI: (A) monoarthritis with swollen, tender joint with decreased range of movements .aspirated material reveals *N. gonorrhoeae* with increased WBC count. Many a times aspirated material may be sterile with raised leukocyte count, (B) another type is of migratory polyarthralgia, of one or two joints with pustular dermatitis, tenosynovitis, may be suppurative.

Q.13 What are other radiological tests are done for evaluation of septic arthritis?

Ans. Ultrasound, radionucleotide imaging, CT scan, and MRI are useful.

Q.14 What is treatment of septic arthritis?

Ans. This should be taken as emergency. As urgent drainage is absolutely necessary under cover of empirical antibiotic therapy and proper antibiotics are started after culture report. After aspiration joint is immobilized and after subsiding of pain passive and active joint movements are started with physical therapy to avoid stiffness.

Q.15 What are methods of draining of joint?

Ans.
- *Needle aspiration* is better for infection of joints not more than 3 days duration, multiple joint affection, and superficial joints easily approachable and the patients who cannot withstand surgery but with thick needle such as of 14-18 gauge as the material is very thick after aspiration joint is lavaged and rested. But if not properly aspirated it may be into chronic infection, needle aspiration cannot be drained completely and thoroughly and in turn more articular cartilage damage and adjacent bone.

- *Open arthrotomy* thorough debridement of joint can be done, proper cleaning of joint, proper savaging can be done, whole joint can be visualized, if there is pannus over articular cartilage it can be cleaned and debrided, all necrotic material can be removed, and then healing is better and prognosis of joint movements is much better after proper rest to the joint.
- *Arthroscopic drainage and lavage* this is minimum traumatizing technique, can be used for every joint except hip, but costly, repeated arthroscopy can be done if needed, with minimum morbidity.

Q.16 What is duration of treatment with intravenous antibiotic?

Ans. Though it is controversial, but should be continued for 2-4 weeks. Now-a-days, it is preferred to start with IV antibiotic for 7-10 days and switched to oral antibiotics after that.

Q.17 What are clinical manifestations of septic bursitis?

Ans. Septic bursitis causes painful swelling in bursa overlying olecranon and patella, which are common sites of septic bursitis. Joint motions are not affected, bit there pain on flexion, due to stretching of overlying tissue, fever may be present (30-40%), skin abrasions, lacerations with sinuses, cellulitis around bursa may be present.

Treatment includes oral or parenteral antibiotics, proper drainage by proper needle aspiration or if not relieved then by open surgical drainage.

CHAPTER 8

Diseases of Elbow

Q.1 What are major types of arthritis of elbow?

Ans. They are rheumatoid, post-traumatic, osteoarthritis (OA) and tuberculosis (TB) of elbow.

Q.2 What are physical findings with elbow arthritis?

Ans. Stiffness of elbow with loss of extension associated with pain in extension and flexion at the extreme range of motion. Bony Crepitus may be palpated with extension/flexion and pronation and supination.

Q.3 What is epidemiology and typical history of elbow arthritis?

Ans. In rheumatology—painful, stiff elbow, with previous diagnosis of rheumatoid arthritis.

Post-traumatic arthritis presents with previous history of fall or trauma to elbow with stiffness, or there is history of heavy labour.

In TB elbow, there is soft doughy fusiform swelling, painful movements, with general signs and symptoms of tuberculosis such as evening rise of temperature, wasting of muscles, with or without sinuses loss of weight, general malaise, etc.

Q.4 What is radiological picture of OA of elbow?

Ans. Anteroposterior (AP) and lateral view of elbow show osteophytes of olecranon and coronoid process and olecranon and coronoid fossae with or without loose bodies. Due to flexion contracture, it is difficult to get real AP view.

Q.5 What is conservative treatment for OA elbow?

Ans.
- Purpose is to relieve pain and to regain or maintain movements.
- Non-steroidal anti-inflammatory drugs, local corticosteroid injection, gentle stretching, may give satisfactory result to some extent.

Q.6 What are surgical procedures are available for OA elbow?

Ans. When there is no satisfactory result obtained after conservative treatment, then also depends upon the extent of stiffness of elbow.
- Capsular release of elbow, removal of loose bodies either by open method or arthroscopically and bony excision if needed such as excision of head of radius, etc.

- Interposition or distraction arthroplasty by ring fixators such as Ilizarao or arthrolysis.
- Synovectomy either by open method or arthroscopically.
- Excisional arthroplasty by interposing some tissues such as skin, membrane, etc.
- Total arthroplasty such as Baxi's implant.
- Open decompression may be done.
- Arthrodesis.

Q.7 What is total arthroplasty?

Ans. When there is replacement of articular surface of lower end of humerus and upper end of ulna with an implant it is called total arthroplasty of elbow. Radial head is not replaced. But trials are being done with silastic radial head (not well established).

Q.8 What are indications of total arthroplasty?

Ans. In cases of advanced elbow arthritis following rheumatoid arthritis, osteoarthritis and post-traumatic arthritis with low demand of function and work. It may be useful in cases of severe communited supracondylar or intercondylar fractures of humerus having stiffness. Or after nonunions of supracondylar fractures in elderly people.

Q.9 What is contraindication for total arthroplasty?

Ans. Infection is absolute contraindication. This operation is not advised in young patients with active life style and heavy laborers.

Q.10 What are types of elbow arthroplasty available?

Ans. *Unlinked or unconstrained:* This resurfaces lower end of humerus and upper ulna with anatomical contours. Stems are attached to improve fixation in the bone. This variety has lowest rate of mechanical loosening but there is instability, dislocation or subluxation so this operation needs very balanced soft tissues.

The fully semiconstrained design-incorporates direct link between ulna and humerus. This allows some dissipation of forces with range of motion at elbow joint. Here the forces are transmitted through the implant-cement-bone interface and this may result in loosening of implant. Fully constrained prosthesis are not used any more semiconstrained design also has loose hinge. This prosthesis has axle and hinge with some rotational laxity in the articulation and allows 10° of varus or valgus. Thus, this semiconstrained has given good results and thus more preferred

Good results are found after both types.

Q.11 What are complications after this operation?

Ans.
- Wound infection,
- Ulnar nerve injury
- Loosening implant
- Instability may be dislocation or subluxation.

Q.12 What are technical considerations of this operation?
Ans.
- Arthroplasty is done usually through posterior approach.
- Proper soft tissue balancing.
- Proper repair of ulnar collateral ligament to avoid instability.

Q.13 What are the results of total arthroplasty?
Ans.
- High satisfaction—with pain relief   90%
- Unsatisfaction   10%
- Long-term results at 10 years   20%

Q.14 What is excision arthroplasty?
Ans. Excision of lower end of humerus with removal of intra-articular osseous parts of elbow joint. Usually done after failed total arthroplasty.

Proper excision of bone of humerus and ulna is very important otherwise it may end up with flail elbow. Some kind of interfacing substance is put between bony ends to avoid reunion then to lead to stiffness again. Such as skin, membrane, etc.

Q.15 What is indication for arthrodesis of elbow?
Ans. It is very difficult to get arthrodesis of elbow. The results are unsatisfactory. No ideal position for fusion of elbow is available and it is done in cases of intractable infection of elbow.

Q.16 What are indications of radial head excision?
Ans. When radiocapitellar joint is involved and ulnohumeral involvement is relatively mild to moderate, then resection of radial head is gives good result as far as pain relief in concerned but without any improvement in movements of elbow. Postoperative movement is variable with 50% unchanged, 30% improved and 20% worse as compared with preoperative movements. This operation does not offer good result in rheumatoid arthritis as this disease is progressive.

Q.17 What is current concept of silastic radial head replacement in elbow surgery?
Ans. Although this operation is recommended by many, but as there is postoperative silicon particulate synovitis and lymphadenitis with subsequent autoimmune response, has decreased its use and not done frequently.

Q.18 What is distraction or interposition arthroplasty? What are its indications?
Ans. It refers to interposing some tissues in between two resected bony ends of elbow. Such as muscle flaps, fascia, skin, gelfoam and fat. External fixators are placed on either side of elbow and then distraction started. This is done in selective patients who do not want arthrodesis or total arthroplasty.

This may not relieve complete pain.

Q.19 What is arthrolysis?

Ans. This is most satisfactory operation for traumatic elbows with myositis ossifications described by Indian orthopaedic surgeon Dr Bhattacharya. This operation includes by taking two incisions on both sides (medial and lateral) joint is opened, dislocated, debris is removed, myositis ossifications is excised and joint is relocated with K-wire fixation, to be removed after 3 weeks followed by vigorous physiotherapy. Very gratifying operation in such cases. There is modification of doing this operation by one incision only that is by lateral incision. Radial head is usually excised.

CHAPTER 9

Supracondylar Fracture of Humerus and Cubitus Varus

Q.1 What is cubitus varus?
Ans. When normal carrying angle of elbow is reduced, then it is called cubitus varus.

Q.2 What is normal carrying angle of elbow?
Ans. In males, it is 10–15° and in females, it is 15–18°.

Q.3 What is cubitus varus?
Ans. When carrying angle is reduced, then it is called cubitus varus.

Q.4 What is cubitus valgus?
Ans. When carrying angle is increased, then it is called cubitus valgus.

Q.5. Why one should treat cubitus varus?
Ans. It is ugly deformity otherwise there is hardly any functional disability.

Q.6 What are causes of cubitus varus?
Ans.
- Malunited supracondylar fracture of humerus
- Congenital
- Malunited lateral condyle fracture of humerus.

Q.7 What is Baumann's angle?
Ans. A perpendicular line is drawn to metaphysoepiphyseal line and another line along axis of humerus and angle which is formed is Baumann's angle which is normally 8–10°.

Q.8 What is three-point relation at elbow?
Ans. In flexed position of elbow, two epicondylar tips, olecranon form isosceles triangle and in extension they are in one line, in normal elbow.

Q.9 What happens in malunited supracondylar fracture to this relation?
Ans. The distance between olecranon tip and two different epicondyles is changed in cubitus varus, it is decreased.

Q.10 What are nerves usually paralysed in supracondylar fractures?
Ans. Two nerves are injured, but most commonly anterior interosseous branch of median nerve, radial nerve tardy, ulnar nerve palsy occurs in cubitus valgus.

Q.11 What is cubitus rectus?
Ans. When there is no valgus or varus angulation.

Q.12 What is shoulder compensation in cases of cubitus varus?
Ans. The coronal tilt-anteroposterior displacement and angulation is compensated at shoulder by internal rotation to keep alignment of elbow normal. There is coronal tilt-varus and anteroposterior displacement—hyperextension at elbow.

Q.13 What are normal movements of elbow?
Ans.
- Flexion 0–145°
- Extension 145–0°
- Supination and pronation at superior radioulnar joint 0–90°

Q.14 How do you treat cubitus varus?
Ans. There is only surgical treatment of corrective osteotomy:
- French osteotomy
- Medial wedge osteotomy
- Modified French osteotomy.

Q.15 What is modified French osteotomy?
Ans. Belmore's modification—two screws are passed first at ends of arms wedge proximally and distally, then wedge is removed and with tension band the angulation is corrected.

Q.16 What are the other osteotomies you know of?
Ans.
- Graziano's osteotomy
- Step-cut osteotomy.

Q.17 What are the features of untreated supracondylar fracture?
Ans.
- Cubitus varus
- Tardy ulnar nerve palsy, if there is cubitus valgus
- Instability of superior radioulnar joint.

Q.18 What is the supracondylar fracture of humerus?
Ans. The fracture of lower end of humerus above the level of olecranon fossa.

Q.19 What are the types of supracondylar fracture of humerus?
Ans.
- Extension type—96%
- Flexion type—4%.

Q.20 What is mechanism of this fracture?
Ans. When there is fall on the ground in hyperextended position of elbow, it is extension type and when there is fall or blow to flexed elbow, it is flexion type.

Q.21 What is classification of supracondylar fracture in children?
Ans. According to Salter and Gartland, they are classified as follows:
Type I: Undisplaced fracture.
Type II: Fracture with angulation or displacement but intact posterior cortex may be with rotational element.
Type III: Completely displaced without any attachment of any cortex. They can be divided again into posteromedial and posterolateral.
One more variety is of where the distal fragment is displaced forward.

Q.22 How do you immobilize these fractures?
Ans. All extension type fractures are to be immobilized in 90° flexion and flexion type in extension. So, it is better to operate these cases and fix with some wires and keep in flexion.

All cases which are done under general anaesthesia, a good traction to be applied for at least 3–5 minutes in extension and then flexion is done with pushing the displaced fragment anteriorly. This is trick for closed reduction.

Q.23 What are complications of supracondylar fracture?
Ans. Malunion–cubitus varus (most common), stiffness of elbow.
- Nerve injuries (5–20%)
- Vascular compromise
- Volkmann's ischemic contracture.

Q.24 What is new approach to treatment of supracondylar fracture?
Ans. Percutaneous pin fixation with help of image intensifier television (IITV) after closed reduction or open reduction and fixation with pin or screws. It should be kept I mind while passing percutaneous pins one has to take care of ulnar nerve on medial side and epiphyseal injuries either medial or lateral.

Q.25 What is mode of pin fixation?
Ans. Two pins are passed after closed reduction on both sides with C-arm control one on medial side and one on lateral side in crossed fashion or two pins are passed in parallel way from lateral side. But crossed pin fixation is more stable. Even pins passed from one point in transeverse V[<] can also give good results.

Q.26 What are indications for open reduction or pin fixation?
Ans.
- Open fractures
- Fractures where closed reduction has failed
- Fractures with vascular complications and nerve complications.

Q.27 What is treatment of medial condyle fracture?
Ans. It depends upon displacement-undisplaced fractures are treated by cast immobilization in flexion for 3-4 weeks. Displaced fracture are to be treated with open reduction and pin fixation it is to be remembered that even minimal displacement has rotational element so they should be treated carefully.

Q.28 Describe treatment of lateral condyle fracture.
Ans. For undisplaced fractures, cast immobilization for 3-4 weeks in flexion. For displaced fractures, open reduction with K-wire fixation is good solution.

Q.29 What are the complications associated with lateral condyle fracture?
Ans. Most common deformity—cubitus valgus. Following malunion, partial growth arrest, or avascular necrosis and nonunion. And tardy ulnar nerve palsy, avascular necrosis of trochlea (fish tail deformity), cubitus varus (rare), lateral spur formation.

Q.30 What is medial epicondyle fracture?
Ans. It is type of avulsion fracture of apophysis in adolescents may follow forced valgus to elbow undisplaced fracture can be treated by complete immobilation and displaced with open reduction with pin fixation.

Q.31 What are the types of supracondylar fractures in adults?
Ans. They are usually direct injuries and they are usually comminuted ones with bag of bones. They are either V-or Y-type and T-shaped fractures. They all are to be treated with pin fixation or with Dunlop traction or with construction plates.

Q.32 What are the complications of these fractures in adults?
Ans. Stiffness of elbow, malunion and nonunion.

10
CHAPTER

Elbow Dislocations and Instability

Q.1 What is dislocation of elbow?
Ans. Dislocation of elbow is defined as dissociation of joint, which connects the humerus with the radius and ulna.

Q.2 What are the types of elbow dislocations?
Ans.
- Posterior or posterolateral—occurs in 90% cases, ulna is posterior to humreus
- Anterior—are rare, associated with high degree of soft-tissue injury
- Lateral
- Medial
- Divergent—though it is rare but quite serious, here radius and ulna dislocate in different directions, here the strong musculocutaneous complex, which binds ulna and radius gets disrupted.

Simple dislocations—dislocations without fracture.
Complex dislocations—dislocations associated with fractures of different components of elbow, making elbow unstable.

Q.3 What are the physical findings in an elbow dislocations?
Ans. Extreme pain, affected forearm is supported by opposite hand in slight flexion, shortening of forearm, palpable olecranon, which is prominent posteriorly with swelling of elbow.

Q.4 What are the fractures associated with dislocation of elbow?
Ans. There are usually—fracture of radial head, coronoid process of ulna, and medial epicondyle.

Q.5 What is the treatment of dislocation of elbow?
Ans. Simple dislocations—without any fracture after checking injury to neurovascular bundle, attempt is to be made to reduce by manipulation to relocate elbow.

Complex dislocation when they are associated with fractures—still closed reduction is attempted, and if not successful then surgery is indicated.

Q.6 What is procedure of reduction of elbow dislocation?
Ans. Reduction is done under either regional or general anaesthesia and should be done immediately to avoid further complications.

- Gentle traction is applied to the forearm with countertraction to distal third of humerus, in supine position of patient and manipulation is done to reduce dislocation.
- With help of assistant who applies steady traction from head side of patient, surgeon applies gentle distal traction to elbow, and elbow is gently extended with correction of medial or lateral deviation, and elbow is flexed and loud chunk is heard indicating that reduction is complete.
- The reduction is done in prone position of patient, gentle downward traction is applied for few minutes and as soon as muscle spasm is released with opposite hand, gentle upward pressure is applied on the distal anterior part of humerus, the arm is lifted keeping traction on, an audible chunk is heard giving ideas of completion of reduction.

A splint or above elbow posterior plaster slab is applied in fully flexed position to be kept for 3-4 weeks and then after removal physiotherapy for movements of elbow started.

Q.7 What is alternative method, if closed reduction fails?
Ans. Open reduction is alternate option after failure of trials of 2-3 closed reductions.

Q.8 What is routine post-reduction treatment?
Ans. There are two views about this:
1. Some advocate immobilising elbow for prolonged period say 3-4 weeks to give time for healing of soft tissue, then starting active and passive movements of elbow without any massage.
2. Since 1986 at USA, there is trend to start active movements as soon as possible instead of immobilising for long time say for one week only to avoid stiffness of elbow, in cases of simple dislocations of elbow.

Q.9 What are the complications of elbow dislocations?
Ans.
- Recurrent dislocations which is very rare.
- Loss of terminal extension of elbow, can be minimised by early range-of-motion programme.
- Heterotopic ossifications may occur.

Q.10 Which ligament is responsible for posterolateral instability of elbow?
Ans. Ulnar portion of lateral collateral ligament is mainly responsible for posterolateral instability of elbow, which results from fall on outstretched hand on the ground. A combination of supination and valgus forces lead to posterolateral instability of elbow.

Q.11 How do you test posterolateral instability of elbow?
Ans. This is tested by lateral pivot test which is done by axial compression, valgus stress and supination. The patient is in supine position and arm is put over the head, examiner is standing at head of table, one hand holds the wrist with forearm in full supination, while other hand is put on the proximal forearm and arm is in full extension, then elbow is slowly flexed with simultaneous axial compression and valgus force to elbow, at 40° of flexion there is feeling of audible chunk by patient or apprehension is indication of positive sign of posterolateral instability of elbow.

CHAPTER 11

Nerve Entrapments of Elbow, Forearm, Wrist and Hand

Q.1 Which is the most common nerve gets compressed in upper extremity?

Ans. The most common nerve gets compressed is median nerve in carpal tunnel syndrome at wrist. Carpal tunnel is formed by carpal bones and roofed by transverse carpal ligament. This is narrow and fibro-osseous rigid canal in which there are nine extrinsic flexors of fingers and thumb with their respective synovial sheaths with median nerve with its sheath carpal tunnel syndrome (CTS) usually seen during middle or advanced age group of females (twice than males), out of which 80% are more than 40 years of age.

Q.2 What is symptomatology of CTS?

Ans. The usual complaint is numbness of fingers, innervated by median nerve (three and half fingers on lateral side). There may be numbness of entire hand, may be some times proximal to wrist, clumsiness or lack of dexterity with the hand due to sensory loss and weakness of thenar muscles. Median nerve is sensory nerve of lateral three and half fingers including thumb and supplies to thenar muscles and two radial lumbrical muscles.

Q.3 What are the common causes of carpal tunnel syndrome?

Ans. Median nerve gets compressed in carpal tunnel due to many reasons, which is decreased in size or increased in volume of contents of the canal.

These are due to pregnancy, rheumatoid arthritis, degenerative arthritis, growth hormone, abnormalities (acromegaly), metabolic (hypothyroidism, gout, diabetes mellitus), alcoholism, tumours, idiopathic, connective tissue disorders (amyloidosis, hemochromatosis), etc.

Q.4 What are the other tests performed to substantiate diagnosis of CTS?

Ans.
- Median nerve percussion test (Tinel's sign)—percussion over median nerve causing paresthesia in the median nerve distribution, then the test is positive.
- Phalen's test-wrist is in full unforced flexion, which increases carpal canal pressure and decreases median nerve blood flow and causing paresthesia or sensory disturbances similar to patient's symptoms for 60 seconds, indicating positive test.

Q.5 What are the other investigations done for diagnosis of CTS?
Ans.
- Laboratory studies to rule out diabetes, gout, renal pathology, thyroid diseases and collagen and vascular diseases.
- X-ray of wrist can reveal fracture, bony spicule, tumor, or arthritis.
- Electrodiagnostic studies—these are sensitive and objective tests to clinch diagnosis of CTS and nerve functions can be assessed before operation.

Q.6 What are the common complications after surgical release of CTS?
Ans. The rate of complications is quite low. But they are—incomplete release of transverse ligament, injury to palmer cutaneous branch or recurrent motor branch of median nerve, reflex sympathetic dystrophy, finger stiffness, decreased strength and persistent tenderness in palmer scar.

Q.7 What is another method of treatment of CTS?
Ans. Part from open surgical release or endoscopic release of CTS can be done with good results and patient can resume his duties earlier with less hospital stay.

Q.8 What is Guyon's canal?
Ans. This is fibro-osseous canal bound by hamate and pisiform bone where the roof is transverse carpal ligament through which ulnar artery and nerve pass without any accompanying tendons.

Q.9 What is the aetiology of neuropathies in Guyon's canal?
Ans. They are trauma, ganglion, lipoma, fracture of hamate and pisiform bone. The common trauma is after bicycling and sensory loss is from distal compression and motor weakness is due to lesion proximal or within canal.

Q.10 What do you mean by Bowler's thumb?
Ans. This traumatic neuropathy of ulnar digital nerve to the thumb may be due to repeated friction or compression of the nerve by edge of thumbhole at bowling ball. The treatment includes adjustment of ball, such as size, shape, spacing, and rarely transposition or neurolysis has to be done for relief.

This can occur in request handball sports. The nerve may be compressed, if there is path near to sesamoid bone.

Q.11 How posterior interosseous nerve compression occurs at wrist?
Ans. Repeated forceful dorsiflexion may irritate this nerve found in gymnastics and rest, splinting, and non-steroidal anti-inflammatory drugs (NSAIDs) can relieve symptoms.

Q.12 How does palmer cutaneous nerve compression occur?
Ans. Blunt trauma can cause transient neuropraxia with symptoms of pain over thenar eminence, may have Tinel's sign positive at edge of transverse carpal ligament. Conservative treatment is more than sufficient.

Q.13 What is double crush syndrome?

Ans. Simultaneous compression of peripheral nerve at multiple locations is called as double crush syndrome. For example, less compression of median nerve is needed at carpal tunnel level to produce symptoms when cervical nerve root compression is present.

Q.14 What is intrinsic plus hand?

Ans. Flexion at metacarpophalangeal joint and extension at interphalangeal joint, and the wrist is held in extension at 10° less than maximal. It is seen in over corrected Bunnel's operation or in rheumatoid arthritis (hand).

Q.15 What is classification of nerve injuries?

Ans. Seddon has classified as follows:
- Neuropraxia—due to localised demyelination from compression or contusion, spontaneous recovery may occur within 2–3 weeks.
- Axonotmesis—due to interruption of axons and their myelin sheath's with intact endoneurial tube may be due to stretching or compression.
- Neurotmesis—due to anatomic disruption of axons, the myelin sheath, and endoneurial tube, due to injury or stretching of the nerve. There may not be automatic recover needs surgical operation such as repair of nerve or nerve grafting, complete recovery is not expected.

Q.16 What is pronator syndrome?

Ans. This is high carpal tunnel syndrome (CTS) as there is entrapment of medial nerve at elbow. Producing numbness, paresthesias in the median nerve innervated digits, weakness of thenar muscles, and pain in the wrist and forearm without any nocturnal symptoms, Tinel's sign is negative at wrist. Causative factor is compression by pronator teres muscle, which can be elicited by resisted forearm pronation with extension of elbow. There may be compression by lacertus fibrosus which is elicited by resisted flexion of elbow with supinated forearm. Sometimes there may be compression by arch of flexor digitorum superficialis which can be tested by resisted flexion of proximal interphalangeal joint of middle finger.

Q.17 What is anterior interosseous syndrome?

Ans. This is compression of anterior interosseous nerve, below 4–6 cm of elbow causing weakness of flexor pollicis longus, flexor digitorum profundus to index and middle fingers and pronator quadratus muscle with pain in forearm.

Q.18 What is cubital tunnel syndrome?

Ans. This referring to entrapment of ulnar nerve during its passage around medial aspect of elbow. Usually, this tunnel is of fibro-osseous ring formed by medial epicondyle and proximal part of the ulna, bridged by special fascial sheet known as Osborne's fascia. Entrapment can occur by repetitive trauma. There may be compression of ulnar nerve, proximal to cubital tunnel due to osteophytes, loose bodies, synovitis, or thickened Osborne's fascia and compression distal to cubital tunnel may occur due to flexor carpi ulnaris aponeurosis or deep flexor pronator aponeurosis, which may be seen in athletes or people with repetitive flexion activities of elbow.

Q.19 How Froment's sign is elicited?
Ans. The patient is asked to pull sheet of paper with index finger and thumb while examiner withdraws it strongly. With normal function of ulnar nerve, the patient maintains maximal contact of digital pulp with paper by extending the IP joint of the thumb but in case of dysfunction of ulnar nerve the control of MP joint is lost due to weakness of the adductor pollicis and deep head of flexor pollicis brevis leading to hyperextension of MCP joint due to its collapse and there is flexion of IP joint to compensate for weakness of pinch.

Q.20 What is radial tunnel syndrome?
Ans. This is also known as resistant tennis elbow is due to entrapment of the posterior interosseous nerve in the lateral aspect of proximal forearm, presenting motor weakness of muscles innervated by radial nerve in the forearm, pain in the lateral aspect of elbow region, or both.

Q.21 What are the structures causing compression of posterior interosseous nerve?
Ans. Fibrous band, recurrent radial vessels, extensor carpi radialis brevis, Arcade of Frose, and supinator are causing compression.

Q.22 What is Wartenberg's syndrome?
Ans. This is entrapment of sensory branch of radial nerve, where it emerges beneath edge of brachioradialis tendon at 6–8 cm proximal to radial styloid and caused by previous trauma or repeated pronation and supination of forearm.

This is shown by inability to adduct extended ring finger which is known as Wartenberg's sign, showing dysfunction of ulnar nerve due to inactivity of the interossei and hypothenar muscles and small finger remains abducted due to unopposed activity of extensor digiti minimi when patient is unable to close V formed by ring and small finger.

CHAPTER 12

Claw Hand due to Hansen's Disease

Q.1 How ulnar nerve is involved in Hansen's disease?
Ans. It is lesion of high ulnar nerve neuritis.

Q.2 What is deformity of hand in Hansen's disease?
Ans. It is claw hand reversal of grasp.

Q.3 What ulnar nerve is frequently affected commonly?
Ans. As it is superficial, has bony bed, low temperature and extensor part of joint moves with every motion.

Q.4 What are different types of leprosy you know off?
Ans.
- Tuberculoid
- Lepromatous

Q.5 What is other classification?
Ans. According to Ridley Jopling,
- Tuberculoid
- Borderline tuberculoid
- Borderline lepromatous
- Lepromatous.

Q.6 What are differential diagnosis of claw hand?
Ans.
- Volkmann's ischemic contracture
- Post-traumatic claw hand.

Q.7 How do you differentiate them?
Ans.
- In leprosy, there are trophic ulcers, sensory involvement, supple hand
- In Volkmann-severe and rigid contracture, no trophic ulcers
- In post-traumatic claw hand-history of trauma, no trophic ulcers and segmental nerve involvement.

Q.8 What is intrinsic minus hand?
Ans. Muscle imbalance with hypoactivity of intrinsic of hand.

Q.9 What is Volkmann contracure?
Ans. Due to soft tissue damage of forearm, there is contracture and paralysis of hand, wrist and forearm (distal half), described by Richard von Volkmann in 1881, which occurs sequelae to compartment syndrome of forearm. There is ischemic muscle damage producing typical deformity of hand and wrist. Extension of fingers can be done when palmer flexion of wrist is done. This is positive Volkmann sign in VIC.

Q.10 What is indication of surgery of decompression of ulnar nerve in Hansen's disease?
Ans. When there is no good recovery after drug therapy and there is bacterial index is less than 1.

Nerve abscess, progressive nerve weakness, consistant pain when there is no good motor function left, and recent and incomplete paralysis of nerve which is not responded to conservative treatment and after steroids which is used for medical decompression.

Q.11 What is lepra reaction?
Ans. Hypersensitivity reactions of two types:
1. Early (within 48 hours)—Fernandez reaction
2. Late (3-4 weeks)—Mistuda reaction

Q.12 What is drug therapy for Hansen's disease?
Ans. *In multibacillary:*
- Rifamycin—600 mg daily for 2 weeks then 600 mg per month
- Dapsone—100 mg daily
- Clofazamine—100 mg on alternate day or 50 mg per day

In paucibacillary:
- Rifamycin—600 mg per month for 6 months
- Dapsone—100 mg per day for 6 months.

Q.13 What are other nerves affected in Hansen's disease?
Ans. Common peroneal nerve:
- Radial nerve
- Median nerve
- Posterior tibial nerve.

Q.14 How will you treat trophic ulcer of foot?
Ans.
- Debridement, nonweight bearing ambulation or ambulation with protection of ulcer by sponge or any such type
- Solution of magnesium sulfate and glycerin with proflavine (MSGP) dressings

- Precautions to avoid injuries
- Keeping local temperature warm.

Q.15 Which is commonly involved nerve?

Ans. Ulnar nerve is most common to get affected (59.9%). There may be combination of nerve affection such a high ulnar and lower median.

Q.16 How operation of decompression is performed?

Ans. Results of decompression are best for ulnar nerve, but even better results have been documented by Dr FH Antia (India).

Epineurium does not allow the expansion of nerve as it is tough, rigid membrane when the edema starts causing pressure from inside. So after exposing nerve at elbow, epineurotomy in longitudinal axis taking care not to damage to blood supply, very much rewarding.

Interfascicular neurolysis is radical surgery where fascicles are dissected and freed from each other, but should not done routinely as this may do further damage to nerve.

Q.17 Is there any other operation in addition to decompression?

Ans. If anterior transposition of ulnar nerve and burying of nerve in bed of common flexor muscles is done with decompression then it gives better result and further damage from repeated trauma due to angulation is prevented.

Q.18 What do you mean by extraneural decompression?

Ans. When medial epicondylectomy by removal of medial epicondyle and medial supracondylar ridge, then the compression over nerve is removed and raw bony surface is covered with muscles.

Olecranon ligament is also cut which is main compressing factor and pivot around which nerve is subjected to repeated trauma with every flexon and extension.

Q.19 Which are tendons available for grafting?

Ans. Plantaris, palmaris longus, fascia lata.

Q.20 How you will treat intrinsic minus hand?

Ans. Paul Brand's tendon transfer—EF4T (Extensor to flexor with four tails)—using extensor carpi radialis longus (ECRL) done in mobile interphalangeal joints.

Bunnel's operation—FF4T (flexor to flexor with four tails) using flexor digitorum sublimis, done in stiff hands with low intelligent quotient patient.

Fowler's operation—extensor digiti minimi and indices are used.

Q.21 How you will overcome loss of opponent's function?

Ans. Flexor digitorum sublimes to ring finger is taken from radial side and transferred to thumb.

Q.22 How tensor fascia lata is useful for grafting?
Ans. It can be easily rolled, has sufficient strength and size.

Q.23 How all tails of tendons are attached and why?
Ans. All tails of tendon of graft are attached on medial border of all fingers except index finger which is attached on lateral side so as to have enhanced adduction of fingers.

Q.24 How do you define claw hand?
Ans. Claw hand follows high or low ulnar nerve palsy where there is paralysis of lumbricales and interossei and other short muscles of hand resulting with variable hyperextension at metacarpophalangeal joints and flexion of proximal and distal interphalangeal joints.

Q.25 Describe grasp mechanism.
Ans. Metacarpophalangeal joints are flexed and interphalangeal joints are extended and tips of fingers are brought together with opposition of thumb this is cupped lumbrical position and thus object is grasped. Metacarpal arch is prominent when cupped lumbrical position is made. It is not possible to perform the act for firm grasping the object or forming bolus of rice or any other objects.

Q.26 What are ways of assessment of deformity of finger joints?
Ans. By—Unassisted angle
 Assisted angle
 Carrying (contracture) angle

Unassisted angle—when the patient is asked to flex his metacarpophalangeal (MP) joint and attempt is made to extend interphalangeal (IP) joint and measured by goniometer. If the angle is large, then there is greater adaptation and with lesser angle less adaptation.

Assisted angle—patient is asked to extend IP joints with support to proximal phalanx. This indicates lack of continuity of dorsal expansion distal to PIP (proximal interphalgeal) joint or there may be anterior displacement of lateral band.

Contracture angle—when attempt is made to extend finger to fullest extent and limitation is measured and thus angle is measured.

Q.27 When tendon transfer is done?
Ans.
- Supple hand
- No infection
- Sufficient muscle power
- No ankylosis of any joints of hand
 By physiotherapy, contracture should be corrected as far as possible.

Q.28 Which are ideal tendons available for grafting?
Ans.
- *Planataris*—advantage-slender, easy removal, easily spillable, and no function is lost after removal, but may absent few cases.
- *Fascia lata*—easy availability, longitudinal fibres, and with variable thickness available.
- *Palmaris longus*—slender, can be easily split, no much function is lost after removal, but may be absent in few cases easily removable.
- *Extensor digitorum to toes*—can be used as free grafts but there may be dropping of toes after removal.

Q.29 What is method of suturing tails to dorsal expansion?
Ans. All tails are sutured to lateral side of expansion except index finger for better pinch, adduction and abduction.

Q.30 What modification of Bunnel to still's operation is required?
Ans. Still was using all tendons of flexor digitorum sublimis which were transferred and attached dorsal expansion thus intrinsic positive hand made by over correction.

Bunnel modified flexor tendon is split into four tails and passed through lumbrical canals to be stitched to dorsal expansion to give better result. Tendon of FDS of ring finger is used most commonly next common is of index finger but as after removal there may be weak pinch and grasp. As FDS of little finger is very weak is not used.

CHAPTER 13

Congenital Disorders

Q.1 What is von Recklinghausen's disease?
Ans. It is neurofibromatosis (NF) with incidence of 1 in 3000 newborns which is autosomal dominant with 50% cases are of spontaneous mutations. Sometimes associated with bilateral acoustic neuroma.

Q.2 What are ways to diagnose neurofibromatosis?
Ans.
- Presence of six or more café au lait maculas at least 5 mm in greatest diameter in prepubertal children and at least 15 mm in greatest diameter in adults
- Two or more neurofibromas of any type or plexiform type
- Optic glioma
- Freckling in the axillary or inguinal regions
- Two or more Lisch nodules (iris hamartomas)
- A clear osseous lesion such as thinning out of cortex of long bones without pseudoarthrosis
- Some other near relative with above criteria may be recognized.

If two or more above criteria are present, then it can be labeled as von Recklinghausen's disease.

Q.3 What are orthopaedic manifestations of NF?
Ans.
- Pseudoarthrosis of long bones usually of tibia but sometimes ulna and clavicles are affected in order of preference. Pseudoarthrosis of tibia starts with anterolateral bowing of tibia in infancy and leading to fracture when child starts walking. Posteromedial angulation is benign and does not lead to fracture
- Scoliosis
- Overgrowth of single digit or whole extremity.

Q.4 What is congenital pseudoarthrosis of tibia?
Ans. Dysplasia of bone and soft tissue with failure of formation of normal bone. Of unknown etiology staring with progressive anterior angulation of tibia and fibula with medullary sclerosis and narrowing of diaphysis or there may be cystic lesion leading to segmental weakening and ultimately pathological fracture. But this not present since birth so it is misnomer. As it develops after birth.

Q.5 What is classification of congenital pseudoarthrosis of tibia?

Ans. Boys and Anderson have classified, based on radiological picture:
- *Dysplastic type*—there is narrowing with sclerosis of tibia may be associated with neurofibromatosis.
- *Cystic type*—after fibrous dysplasia with good prognosis
- *Sclerotic type*—there is sclerosis without narrowing
- *Early type*—pseudoarthrosis present at birth.

Q.6 What are goals of treatment?

Ans. To obtain union, maintain union, correct deformity, and obtain limb length equality.

Q.7 What are principles of treatment of congenital pseudoarthrosis of tibia?

Ans. The principle is excision of dysplastic segment followed by use of autologous grafts.

The following methods have proved quite successful:
- *Intramedullary rod*—corrects deformity, prevent refracture, easy to do, but limb equality is not achieved
- *Vascular fibular graft*—very specialised technique, but with high rate of success and add some length of limb
- *Ilizarov technique*—allows compression of pseudoarthrosis and lengthening is done but there is high risk of refracture

Recent studies have shown that Ilizarov with IM rod has given good results without risk of refracture.

Q.8 What is treatment of pseudoarthrosis of tibia?

Ans.
- Spontaneous union is extremely rare
- Bracing or casting can be used to start with as palliative method
- Plating with bone grafting—success rate is 50%
- Free vascularized bone grafts with external fixator (such as Illizarao) or intramedullary rod.
- *Seekh kabab* operations such as multiple osteotomies with intramedullary rod
- Amputation either below knee or Syme's amputation, if all other procedures fail.

Multiple operations are needed to get successful result but may lead to shortening, angulation, and stiffness of joints.

Q.9 When amputation is indicated for congenital pseudoarthrosis of tibia and of what type?

Ans. When repeated surgeries fail to unite and when there is ankle stiffness, or severe deformity and shortening. Amputation is indicated.

Ankle disarticulation (Boyd and Syme operation) is advised rather than amputation through the lesion as it avoids problems of spike formation and provide good end bearing skin and gives some length also.

Q.10 What are other causes of pseudoarthrosis of tibia?
Ans.
- Fibrous dysplasia
- Trauma—old compound fracture of tibia
- Infection—infected nonunion of tibia.

Q.11 What is arthrogryposis?
Ans. Arthrogryposis is group of nongenetic congenital contracture syndromes of unknown origin characterized by affection of both upper extremities, which are addicted and internally rotated, at shoulder, elbows are extended and wrists an fingers are flexed, with thumb in palm, lower extremities are flexion, abducted, and externally rotated hips, knees may be flexed or extended and clubfeet may be associated. They are rigid and resistant to treatment.

Q.12 What is Klippel-Feil syndrome?
Ans. Klippel-Feil (KF) syndrome is group of deformities that result from failure of segmentation of cervical vertebrae. Patients have low posterior hair line, short neck, limited cervical spine movements especially lateral bending, and may be associated with Sprengel's deformity, scoliosis, abnormalities of urinary tract, congenital heart disease, with loss of hearing.

Q.13 What is Sprengel's deformity?
Ans. This is characterized by an elevated and rotated scapula, due to stoppage of caudal migration of scapula may be bound by fibrous tissue, cartilage, or an omovertebral bone to cervical spine. All patients with KF syndrome have loss of abduction and forward flexion. Physiotherapy of stretching type exercises usually do not help so the treatment of choice is surgery.

ARTHROGRYPOSIS MULTIPLEX CONGENITA

Q.1 What is arthrogryposis multiplex congenital?
Ans. This is nonprogressive congenital disorder where there are multiple joint contractures, which is diagnosed by an exclusion method.

Q.2 What is typical clinical picture of arthrogryposis multiplex congenital?
Ans. The extremities are of tubular shape, with absent skin creases and they are in either extension or flexion joint contractures.

Q.3 What is classification of this disease?
Ans.
  A. *Quadrimelic*—where all four limbs are involved
  B. *Bimelic*—where upper or lower two limbs are affected (most common)
  C. *Monomelic*—where only one limb is involved.

Congenital Disorders **43**

Q.4 What are clinical features to diagnose?

Ans. The diagnosis is made by clinical picture of typical positions of multiple joints such as:
- The shoulders are addicted and internally rotated with weakness of deltoid muscle
- Extension contracture of elbow due to weakness of biceps and brachialis
- Wrist is flexed with ulnar deviation due to contracture of flexor carpi ulnaris
- The thumb is addicted with thumb in palm position due to contracture of adductor pollicis and 1st web contracture with typical flexion of fingers at metacarpophalangeal, proximal interphalangeal and distal interphalangeal joints with limitation of active and passive movements
- Hip dysplasia or dislocation with flexion, abduction and external rotation contracture
- Flexion deformity of knee due to weakness of quadriceps muscle
- Clubfoot (Congenital talipes equinovarus) sometimes with vertical talus or calcaneovalgus deformity of foot
- Sometimes there may be micrognathia and microstomia with facial midline hemangioma
- There may be labial hypoplasia in females and inguinal hernias in males.

Q.5 What is other way of classification of arthrogryposis multiplex congenital?

Ans. They are:
- Neuropathic—there is dysfunction of anterior horn cells, which is most common, 95%
- Myopathic, where muscles are affected—5%

Q.6 What is typical histopathology of muscle in neuropathic form?

Ans. Muscles are denervated, and partially replaced by fat and fibrous tissue, increase in neuromuscular junctions, fiber type disproportion, in remaining muscle tissue, increase in collagen tissue leading periarticular fibrosis and causing joint contracutres.

Q.7 What are general concepts in treatment of arthrogryposis?

Ans.
- Physical and occupational therapy
- Use of proper orthotics
- Surgery—release of soft tissues which is done at early age and osteotomies at later age, such as in childhood and adolescents, to correct deformities and joint contractures.

Q.8 What different modalities of surgery at different regions?

Ans. The contractures are rigid and quite resistant to treatment.
- *Shoulder*—adduction and internal rotation deformity causes minimal functional disability, so no active treatment is needed, except derotational osteotomy of humerus can be done in extreme cases.

- *Elbow*—for extension contracture-posterior capsulotomy with or without muscle or tendon transfer such as triceps, pectoralis major latissimus dorsi to the biceps to get better functional results. Sometimes derotational osteotomy of humerus done for very stiff elbow.
- *Wrist*—for flexion and ulnar deviation-serial casting and splinting for infants. Volar capsulotomy with transfer of tendon of flexor carpi ulnar is to extensor carpi radialis for young children, sometimes carpectomy or wrist fusion is advised in adolescents and adults.
- *Thumb*—lengthening of adductor pollicis and deepening of 1st webspace, volar release with skin grafting, occasional arthrodesis.
- *Hip*—extensive open reduction with or without derotation osteotomy of femur is done which is controversial
- *Knee*—for flexion contractures-posterior knee capsulotomy with release of hamstrings muscles. Ilizarov frame or Joshi's external stabilization system (JESS) fixator is more useful. Some advise supracondylar osteotomy. Extension contracture does not need treatment
- *Foot*—clubfeet has to be treated surgically with JESS fixator or ilizarov frame as these deformities are recurrent or extensive soft tissue release, talectomy, are done to overcome recurrences.

DEVELOPMENTAL DYSPLASIA OF HIP

Q.1 What is developmental dysplasia of hip (DDH)?

Ans. This is progressive condition of hip where hip structures do not develop normally.

Three stages are there as follows:
1. Head of femur is in the normal acetabulum with minimal physical findings.
2. Head moved slightly away from medial wall of acetabulum.
3. Head of femur has moved out of acetabulum.

First two stages are supposed to be precursor of dislocation.

Q.2 What are types of DDH?
Ans.
- *The dislocated hip*—the hip is dislocated, in resting position as there is no contact between the femoral head cartilage and acetabulum.
- *The dislocatable hip*—hip can be dislocated during examination but not dislocated at rest
- *The subluxatable hip*—the hip is not dislocated at rest but can be subluxated partial dislocation-partial contact between head
- *The dysplastic hip*—no signs of instability, the femoral head and acetabulum are abnormally shaped and developed.

Congenital Disorders

Q.3 What are Ortolani's and Barlow's test? What is significance?

Ans. *Ortolani's test*: This is to test instability of hip by stress maneuvers, positive test signifies that the dislocated hip is reducible, the patient is supine, with flexion of knee, with thumb of hand on medial side and other fingers on greater trochanter, with support to pelvis, the hip is brought from midline in 90° flexion and is abducted, with gentle lifting of greater trochanter, the head shifts into acetabulum and the sensation of this reduction is appreciated in cases of dislocated hips. This is positive sign.

Barlow's test: This tests identifies that the hip is dislocatable or subluxatable. The patient is supine, hip is flexed at 90^0 and is brought from abduction to adduction and just beyond neutral abduction a gentle posterior pressure is applied to the thigh. The sensation of femoral head moving posteriorly out of socket indicates positive Barlow's test.

Q.4 What is Galeazzi sign with what significance?

Ans. This is for evaluation of apparent length of thigh. The patient is supine, with thighs held together and raised to 90° hip and knee flexion position and level of knees is evaluated and any shortening is assessed. In unilateral affection, it is obvious but both knees are at equal level in bilateral affection.

Q.5 What is role of plain X-ray in DDH?

Ans. Anteroposterior view is taken with extended hips with neutral rotation, and following inferences are drawn—DDH shows delayed femoral ossification, discontinuity of Shenton's line, increased acetabular index (angle between Hilgenreiner's line and line drawn parallel to the acetabulum) compared with normal hip.

Based on this findings, DDH can be reliably diagnosed.

Q.6 Does ultrasound play any significant role?

Ans. Yes, ultrasound can provide details of femoral head and acetabular configuration below the age of 6 months. Additional information can be done with use of pelvic harness (orthosis). This gives better information than plain X-ray.

Q.7 What is treatment of newborn of DDH?

Ans. The treatment with pelvic harness is treatment of choice for the child with dislocated, dislocatable or subluxatable hip. Even this harness is applied at the time of diagnosis and used for 8-12 weeks for hip to become stable in unstable hip, below the age of 6 months.

Q.8 What is Pavlik harness?

Ans. It is flexion-abduction orthosis consisting of chest strap, anterior flexion straps, posterior abduction straps to maintain affected limb in 90°-100° of flexion to limit abduction, being not rigid device, child's own muscles help to maintain the hip in reduced position. This gives success in 90-95% cases below the age of 6 months.

Q.9 What is treatment of DDH in 6-18 months old child?
Ans. Closed reduction is attempted after skin traction for short period and maintained by hip spica for one and half limb with or without adductor tenotomy.

Q.10 What are indications of open reduction for DDH?
Ans. When closed reduction fails, open reduction by medial or anterolateral approach with femoral shortening procedures, is the treatment of choice for children older than 2 years.

Q.11 What are other methods of treatment of DDH or CDH?
Ans.
- *Salter's innominate osteotomy*—is pelvic cut made from sciatic notch to just below the anterior superior iliac spine, acetabulum is hinged anteriorly and laterally pivoting on the pubic symphysis and displacement is maintained by wedge of iliac crest bone graft and may be fixed with pins indicated in cases of mild to moderate acetabular dysplasia to increase stability.
- *Pemberton osteotomy*—indicated in severe acetabular dysplasia, when not corrected by Salter's osteotomy. The ilium is cut to triradiate cartilage, acetabulum is hinged anteriorly and laterally on flexible cartilage and wedge of iliac crest is inserted to maintain the displacement.
- *The steel triple innominate osteotomy*—indicated in older children and with severe dysplasia who had minimal mobility at pubic symphysis or triradiate cartilage. The ilium is cut similar way of Salter's osteotomy, two additional cuts are taken, one through ischium and another through superior pubic ramus, entire acetabulum is rotated in such way to provide good acetabular coverage to femoral head.
- The Ganz osteotomy—is similar to Steel operation, with similar indications and it is done through only one incision and cuts leave posterior and pelvis intact.
- The Chiari osteotomy—indicated in severe dysplastic cases, oblique cut is made through ilium at level of anterior inferior iliac spine, acetabulum is displaced medially, when ilium abuts superior and lateral capsule and acts as shelf to cover lateral aspect of uncovered and subluxated femoral head.
- Shelf operation iliac crest bone grafts are pushed into lateral aspect of ilium at the level of acetabular margin, is indicated in hips with residual dysplasia with uncovered femoral head and where congruous reduction of hip is not achieved by other osteotomies.

Q.12 What are complications of DDH when untreated?
Ans.
- In unilateral cases, there will be limb length discrepancy with Trendelenburg type limp
- Though painless movements but early onset of osteoarthritis of hip

- In bilateral cases—patients walk with extension of lumbosacral spine-hyperlordosis with high rock of OA of hip
- Proximal femoral growth disturbances when untreated to treatment has failed.

Q.13 What are other options of treatment for residual DDH or subluxated hip in adolescents and young adults?
Ans.
- Redirectional pelvic osteotomy can be done for coverage of femoral head
- With pelvic osteotomy femoral osteotomy can be done for better results
- In cases of incongruent and deficient lateral coverage over femoral head, the shelf or Chiari operation may give better result with advanced OA of hip and acetabular dysplasia or subluxation, hip fusion in adolescents or surface arthroplasty or total arthroplasty is done.

SKELETAL DYSPLASIA

Q.1 Who is pioneer person for skeletal dysplasia?
Ans. Sir Thomas Fairbank of Edinburgh, Scotland in 1951 by writing his book on An Atlas of General Affections of Skeleton.

Q.2 What are definitions of dysplasia, dwarfism, midget, dysostosis, and deformity?
Ans. Dysplasia—there are generalized developmental changes in the skeleton.
Dwarfism—pathologic diminution in stature, divided into:
- Midget—proportionate dwarfism
- Disproportionate—short limb—again subdivided into:
  Rhizomelic—proximal portion is shortened
  Mesomelic—middle portion is short
  Acromelic—distal portion is short
- Dysostosis—developmental changes of single bone or segment of the skeleton
- Malformation—primary abnormality of development
- Deformity—changes in previous normal bone.

Q.3 What is multiple epiphyseal dysplasia (MED)?
Ans. There are irregularities in development of epiphysis leading to late appearance of or mottling of ossification a center, knobby joints stubby digits, minor shortening of stature with or without vertebral involvement.

Q.4 What is chondrodysplasia?
Ans. There is stippling of epiphysis, disordered longitudinal bone growth, mental retardation, and cataract.

Q.5 What is Stickler's syndrome?

Ans. There are changes of epiphysis similar to MED, severe progressive myopia, with retinal detachment and blindness, hearing loss, cleft palate, spinal deformities, such as anterior wedging and spinal scoliosis.

Q.6 What is most common type of dwarfism?

Ans. The most common type is achondroplasia with short limbed disproportionate disorder resulting from defective formation of enchondral bone. Clinical picture is as follows: short limbs, large bulging cranium, low nasal bridge, narrowed spinal canal in lumbar region, with pelvic changes, thoracolumbar kyphosis, or lumbar canal stenosis.

Q.7 Can lengthening or correction of angular deformity be done in skeletal dysplasia cases?

Ans.
- By using callus distraction (callotasis) surgical technique there can be gain in length up to 7 cm in femur and tibia with good function but malalignment of mechanical axis of the bones. With higher percentage of complications as compared to normal children.
- Correction of angular deformities such as genu varum can be achieved by hemichondrodiatasis where distraction is applied through only portion of growth plate (physis).

Q.8 What is marble bone disease?

Ans. This is also called osteopetrosis where there is failure of bone resorption due to functional deficiency of osteoclasts with persistence of calcified chondroid and primitive bone. On X-ray, there are opacities of bone with lack of cortical endosteal margins and failure of bone remodeling. Only treatment is marrow transplantation.

Q.9 What is spotted bone disease?

Ans. This is also called Osteopoikilosis where dense ovoid or circular spots are seen in cancellous bone, found in clusters in metaphyseal or epiphyseal regions of long bones, not affecting cortex or contour of bone, may be present since birth usually located at carpal, tarsal, bones, end of large tubular bones, or around acetabulum causing no symptoms and hence no treatment is needed.

Q.10 What is Caffey's disease?

Ans. This also called infantile hyperostosis with findings such as swelling of soft tissues, cortical thickening of underlying bone with hyperirritability Though this was described first by Roske in 1930 but thoroughly studied and described by Caffey and Siverman in 1945.

Q.11 What is osteogenesis imperfect (OI)?

Ans. This is several genetically and clinically heterogenous syndromes consisting of skeletal gracility with blue sclera, deafness, and hyperlaxity of ligaments with clinical picture of multiple fractures, knee deformities and scoliosis.

Q.12 What is Marfan's syndrome?

Ans. This is characterized by disproportionate long, thin limbs and digits, scoliosis, generalized joint laxity, dislocation of lens, dissecting aortic aneurysm, prolapsed cardiac valves, and prevalence of hernias, Marfan was French pediatrician who described this condition.

Q.13 What is Ehlers-Danlos syndrome (ED)?

Ans. ED is group of syndromes caused by defective collagen metabolism and having clinical picture of skin changes of hyperextensibility, fragility, and easy bruisability with resultant cigarette paper scarring, extreme ligamentous laxity of joints, bone fragility with osteopenia has no specific treatment.

Q.14 What are dyschondroplasia, Ollier's disease, and Maffucci's syndrome?

Ans.
- *Dyschondroplasia*—rare disease with circumscribed masses of cartilage arranged in linear fashion in the interior of bone.
- *Ollier's disease*—multiple enchondromas due to hamartomatous proliferation of cartilage cells originating within the bones and from cambium layer of periosteum. When the lesion is unilateral is called Ollier's disease.
- *Maffucci's syndrome*—multiple enchondromas with multiple hemangiomas, need good monitoring of the patient such as Ollier's disease.

CHAPTER 14

Clubfoot

CONGENITAL TALIPES EQUINOVARUS

Q.1 What is CTEV?

Ans. It is congenital talipes equinovarus foot.

Q.2 What are types of CTEV?

Ans.
- Congenital
  - Idiopathic
  - Associated with other congenital conditions such as spina bifida, meningocele, myelocoele, etc. congenital absence of tibia and growing fibula.
- Acquired

Q.3 What are theories of idiopathic CTEV?

Ans. There are few theories for this condition:
- Trauma during pregnancy (esp. 1st trimester)
- Radiation exposure during pregnancy
- Ingestion of toxic drugs during pregnancy such as thalidomide
- Dr Duraiyaswami's insulin theory by giving fractions of insulin one can produce many deformities
- Attack of German rubella during pregnancy
- Infection.

Q.4 What are reasons of acquired CTEV?

Ans.
- Following poliomyelitis
- Musculogenic—such as muscular dystrophy, associated with arthrogryposis fetalis where defect is with muscle cell
- Neurogenic—in conditions such as cerebral palsy, spina bifida ocular, etc.
- Following trauma such as loss of medial pillar of leg, i.e. tibia or its part
- Congenital absence of tibia or its part
- Overgrowth of fibula.

Q.5 What are types of CTEV as per condition of foot?
Ans.
- Supple
- Rigid
- Resistant
- Neglected
- Relapsed.

Q.6 What are deformities in CTEV?
Ans.
- Varus of forefoot
- Caves at midfoot
- Inversion of hindfoot.

Q.7 How do you grade CTEV?
Ans.
- Mild—where deformity can be easily corrected
- Moderate—where deformity can be corrected with gentle force under anesthesia
- Severe—where the deformity can not be corrected even under anesthesia, the medial border of great toe is touching medial border of tibia.

Q.8 What are bad prognostic signs?
Ans.
- Small inverted heel
- Severe cavus at midfoot (folding of forefoot on hindfoot at midfoot)
- Severe forefoot varus
- In cases of arthrogryposis
- Good callosity on lateral side of foot.

Q.9 What is shape of foot in clubfoot?
Ans. There is convexity on lateral side and concavity on medial side.

Q.10 How does child walks?
Ans. The child when stars walking walks on lateral border of foot and with elevated heel. That is why there are callosities on lateral side of foot.

Q.11 Where are major deformities?
Ans. At subtalar joint and talonavicular joint complex.

Q.12 As per Le Noir's hypothesis to which joint what deformity occurs?
Ans. Equinaus at ankle, inversion at subtalar joint, adduction at Chopart and Lisfranc's joint.

Q.13 When one should start treatment?
Ans. Immediately one can start just after birth but the skin is very soft so one has to wait at least for three weeks.

Q.14 What are ways?

Ans. Gentle manipulation should be started by mother herself while giving bath taking care not to injure lower epiphysis of tibia [so she should hold firmly lower end of tibia] and slowly and gradually and gently manipulate the foot into eversion many times. Tickling on lateral side by blunt object such as pencil or pen so that child tries to do eversion of foot to correct varus deformity.

Q.15 What are methods of conservative treatment?

Ans.
- Manipulation
- Strapping by adhesive plaster
- POP cast after manipulation under GA
- Plaster slabs and wedging.

Q.16 How strapping is done?

Ans. After three weeks of life strapping is done. At least 2–3 times week, over and above each strapping and giving one holiday, i.e. Monday to Saturday and on Sunday the foot is left without strapping for cleaning and washing the foot and leg. This is done for 3–4 months to make the foot supple so as to avoid major operation if possible.

Q.17 How strapping should be done?

Ans. Strapping should be started from inwards to outwards, i.e. from medial side of addicted foot to sole of foot, then taking turn to lateral side of foot and leg to medial side of knee and leg (take care of peroneal nerve at fibular head by putting small cotton pad and even pads are to be kept on all bony prominences) by extra porous (preferably) adhesive plaster and then by bandage over it. Spoiling by urine, can be taken care by putting foot and leg in plastic protective bag.

Q.18 How does strapping helps?

Ans. Every time when child kicks the foot goes into valgus and helps in correcting deformity, thus dynamically correction occurs. It helps in retention of muscle power and tone.

Q.19 What are complications of strapping?

Ans. Allergy to adhesive plaster, care is taken by application of lactocalamine such as medicines.
- Skin ulcers
- Peeling of skin.

Q.20 How POP cast is applied? What are precautions to be taken?

Ans. Under full general anesthesia gently manipulation is done, maintained and above knee pop cast is applied by keeping knee in 90° flexion. Care is taken to strengthen medial side of plaster of foot. Care of bony prominences is taken by keeping good padding to avoid ulceration. Reduced position is maintained till cast is set properly.

The manipulation should be gently as forcible manipulation may cause petechial hemorrhages and that may cause fibrosis and foot may become more rigid.

Q.21 How often and how long one should continue POP cast method?
Ans. It should be done once a month, if plaster is intact or not broken.

One can continue pop cast method for 3-4 months, by changing plaster once a month. This is good initial method for patients who are coming from long distance or so those who can not come oftenly for strapping.

Q.22 Which deformity recurs first of clubfoot?
Ans. Equinus.

Q.23 Which are structures are tight on medial side?
Ans.
 A. Longus abductor hallucis longus
 B. Ligaments—Deltoid ligament, spring ligament, capsule of subtalar joint, end of talonavicular joint.

Q.24 How do you select patient for surgery?
Ans. One has to assess about rigidity, recurrency, relapsing residual deformity, and neglected and size of foot then one has to opt for surgery.

Q.25 What are types of surgeries you know of for clubfoot in children?
Ans.
- Soft tissue operations—posterior release, posteromedial release, complete subtalar release, tarsometatarsal capsulotomy if not sufficient all together called soft tissue release
- Bony operations in children before age of maturity, Calcaneal osteotomy (Dwayer), talar neck
- Evans operation-excision of bone from cuboid.

Q.26 What are surgeries after age of maturity?
Ans. Triple arthodesis.

Q.27 What is postoperative regime after soft tissue release?
Ans. Immediate above knee pop cast after correction, which is done as much as possible. If there is vascular compression or so then full correction is not done after 2-3 weeks sutures are removed and pop cast applied after full correction. Knees are kept on 90^0 flexion to avoid slipping of plaster cast.

Q.28 What is Turco's procedure?
Ans. Internal fixation with K wire is used after posteromedial release.

Q.29 Who are Indian orthopaedic surgeons who have contributed work on clubfoot?

Ans.
- Dr B Mukhopadhyay—Patna procedure complete soft tissue release.
- Dr RL Mittal—Rotational skin flap reconstruction to correct posteromedial skin contractures.
- Dr BB Joshi—New external fixator known as JESS.

Q.30 What is Rocker bottom foot?

Ans. Vertical talus with equines hind foot and forefoot is dorsiflexed and midfoot is down like soccer, may be after improper treatment or complication of inadequate treatment.

Q.31 What is recent treatment for CTEV?

Ans. Dr BB Joshi has devised external fixator called JESS which can be applied even in children. Ilizarov ring fixator—which is rather cumbersome than JESS.

Q.32 What are advantages?

Ans. This can be done even in children before age of maturity very useful in rigid and neglected clubfoot. The size of foot remains normal. Less complications, easy to handle, no big operative scars, recurrence rate is very low.

Q.33 What is JESS?

Ans. Joshi's controlled external stabilizing system (differential distraction).

Q.34 What is time limit to continue treatment?

Ans. Till child starts walking like normal foot.

Q.35 How long one should follow patient?

Ans. There is always fear of recurrence or relapse. So ideally the patient should be followed till the age of maturity.

Q.36 Is any tendon transfer needed?

Ans. If at all needed one has to transfer of tendon of tibialis anterior to medial cuneiform, if there is no proper correction in spite of all other surgeries.

CHAPTER 15

Foot Drop

Q.1 What is the cause of foot drop in Hansen's lesion?
Ans. Usually the common peroneal nerve is involved before branching and affected in toto.

Sometimes the paralysis is incomplete as there is involvement of anterior tibial nerve causing loss of dorsiflexion. But when common peroneal nerve is involved, there is loss of dorsiflexors and evertors leading to complete foot drop especially. Foot drop in addition to equines position may cause ulceration on lateral border to the foot.

Q.2 What do you mean by established foot drop?
Ans. Foot drop lasting for more than one year, which is resistant to conservative treatment.

Q.3 What is important thing to be taken care of?
Ans. When there is established foot drop, then only one can think of doing tendon transfer or some operative procedure.

Q.4 What is the difference between foot drop of polio and after Hansen's disease?
Ans. There are no sensory changes in polio and persistent equines deformity seen in polio. The foot is plantigrade in Hansen foot drop and high steppage gait.

Q.5 What are muscle transfers done for foot drop?
Ans. Tibialis posterior is transferred either through interosseous membrane or circumtibial way to dorsum of foot to replace the action of tibialis anterior.

Q.6 Describe the care taken in this operation.
Ans. The tendon should be transferred with proper mechanical advantage when passed around tibia.

Care to be taken not to injure metatarsal bones or may be sutured to dorsiflexors to avoid fracture.

Q.7 What physiotherapy is done postoperatively?
Ans. Physiotherapy should be started even before surgery to educate the patient how to use tibialis posterior to elevate foot.

Tibialis posterior stabilizes subtalar joints during weight bearing but order of elevation of foot takes some time as it is related to lumbar segments 4 and 6. Passive stretching is also taught.

CHAPTER 16

Evaluation of Hip Disease

It will be a long case in the examination so it is important to take detailed history and must have detailed description, such as what type of pain is there, does this radiate and how? Whether pain is more at night, etc. One should inquire about limp, history of any trauma, etc.

After this, one should start inspection, and under this heading, one should see attitude, then one should confirm the points of inspection and then one can proceed to movements, special tests, measurements and one should evaluate the other hip and knee. You have got sufficient time for detailed examination. Please remember that once you have completed examination, you should not touch again and you should demonstrate all special tests and measurements to examiner in his presence and try to convince him. You should be perfect in clinical tests, measurements and special tests.

There are few commonly asked questions in practical examination.

Q.1 What is range of movements of normal hip joint?
Ans.
- Extension 0°
- Flexion 120°
- Abduction 45°
- Adduction 30°
- External rotation 45° and internal rotation 45°.

Q.2 Why patient of affected hip complains pain in knee and anterior to thigh?
Ans. Due to common nerve supply by femoral and obturator nerve.

Q.3 Why is there increased lumbar lordosis?
Ans. Physiological causes—pregnancy, obesity
Pathological causes—due to fixed flexion deformity in TB hip, bilateral dysplasia of the hip (CDH).

Q.4 What are the conditions where you get asymmetry of gluteal folds seen from back?
Ans. May be due to CDH, muscular dystrophy, pelvic obliquity, inequality of lengths of limbs.

Q.5 What is pelvic obliquity?

Ans. When two anterior iliac spines are not at same level, it is concluded that pelvis is oblique. This may be due to scoliosis or contracture of hip (commonly) adduction and flexion.

Q.6 How is Thomas test done?

Ans. This test is done for assessment of flexion contracture of the affected hip. The patient is made to lie on table or hard bed, normal limb is flexed at hip and knee so as to touch anterior surface of thigh to anterior surface of abdomen and chest and held and maintained by the patient himself, then the lordosis, which is created by affected hip has to be obliterated so that hand cannot be passed underneath back, an attempt is made to extend the limb with little force and then angle which is formed by ground to flexed limb is the angle of flexion of contracture. And with stabilizing pelvis, free flexion is measured after this angle and assessed accordingly.

Q.7 When do you get false-positive Thomas test?

Ans. In scoliosis and polio due to pelvic obliquity, exaggerated lordosis due to pregnancy, postural abnormalities, spondylolisthesis, etc.

Q.8 How flexion contracture is measured when both hips are affected?

Ans. This is best measured in prone position the patient is made to lie on couch and asked to support his knees on the examiner's hand and gradually limb is extended and the point of resistance is reached and the angle is measured between the trunk and thigh.

In supine position, both limbs are lifted till disappearance of lordosis and angle is measured which is angle of flexion deformity.

Q.9 What is Trendelenburg's test?

Ans. This test gives idea about gluteus medius muscle. This test can be done from back and from the front.

When seen from the back, affected limb is lifted up and the level of gluteal fold is elevated due to normal contraction of gluteal muscle but when patient is standing on affected limb and normal limb is lifted up, due to weakness of gluteal muscle, pelvis sags down and level of fold is lower than normal. This indicated positive Trendelenburg test. This is due to nonfunctioning or weak gluteus medius muscle or the link lever with fulcrum-neck, lever arm of abductors is lost such as nonunion of fracture neck of femur or so.

Q.10 What are the conditions where Trendelenburg test is positive?

Ans.
- In sufficiency of gluteus medius muscle—fracture neck of femur (old), coax vara, CDH, Perthe's disease, etc.
- Gluteal paralysis—following polio, muscular dystrophy, motor neuron disease, flaccid cerebral palsy.
- Gluteal apprehension—pain from hip diseases.

Q.11 What is gradation of Trendelenburg test?
Ans.
- Grade I—30 seconds
- Grade II—45 seconds
- Grade III—60 seconds.

Q.12 When Trendelenburg test cannot be done?
Ans. This test cannot be done in the following conditions—When patient cannot stand and bear weight, when there is ankylosis of hip due to any reason, when there is any residual deformity such as adduction or abduction, and when the patient cannot lift limb more than 30°.

Q.13 How do you account for hip limp?
Ans. During midstance, the hip is displaced laterally by one inch then to weight bearing side; but with hip limp, the lateral displacement is accentuated resulting in exaggerated limp.

Q.14 What is common abnormality of CDH?
Ans. There is adduction contracture with 90° flexion in bilateral CDH, but there is shortening in unilateral dislocation.

Q.15 What is typical physical abnormality in slipped capital femoral epiphysis?
Ans. There is increased external rotation with diminished internal rotation due to displacement of femoral head to posterior and inferior direction.

Q.16 What is figure four-test? What are other names for that?
Ans. While the patient is in supine position, examiner flexes, externally rotates and abducts hip so as to place heel over uninvolved knee and the patient with hip pathology has diminished range of motion of hip or unable to do this maneuver or do so without significant pain.

This is also called Patrick's test and FABER test, which is apprehension test and indicates anterior labral tear.

Q.17 What is Ely's test? What inference does it give?
Ans. This is for contracture of rectus femoris. The patient is made to lie in prone position, then knee is flexed to 90° and if hip on same side also gets spontaneous flexion, then there is contracure of rectus femoris on that side. If not affected, then the patient remains flat on the bed or in neutral position.

Q.18 What is Ober's test?
Ans. This is for assessment of contracture of iliotibial band. The patient is made to lie on unaffected side, the leg is slowly abducted with extended hip with flexion of knee to 90°, the leg is slowly released and from abduction to neutral position, in cases of contracture of iliotibial band, the thigh remains in abducted position.

Q.19 What is telescopic test? What is its significance?

Ans. The patient is taken on hard bed, hip and knee are flexed to 90°, limb is adducted to 5°–15°, by securing hand posteriorly and over trochanter—push and pull, manoeuvre is done to feel recoil over the hand. It is present in CDH, old dislocations, pathological dislocations, non-union fracture neck of femur, after excision arthroplasty of hip.

In post-traumatic cases, one may get crepitus in addition to this.

Q.20 What is false-negative and false-positive telescopic test?

Ans.
- When limb is in abduction, the test is negative
- When there is joint laxity and soft bed, one can get false-positive test.

Q.21 Is aspiration useful in hip pathology?

Ans. Hip aspiration is very much useful in differentiating septic arthritis and transient synovitis. But wide bore needle should be used, say 16 or 14 number. It may be useful in assessment of infection after surgery such as hemiarthroplasty, or total hip replacement (THR), analysis of synovial fluid and then local, injections if needed can be given.

Q.22 How tomography is useful for hip?

Ans. It is useful in trauma cases, especially nonunion of fracture neck of femur, internal fixation devices, for any loose bone piece after reduction of dislocated hip, to know configuration of acetabulum, evaluation of stress femoral neck fractures. Plain tomography is more useful when computed tomography (CT) is not available.

Q.23 What advantages do you get from CT scan of hip and pelvis?

Ans. CT scan is very effective in traumatic conditions especially delineating fracture line of iliac crest, acetabulum, sacrum, to evaluate any loose bony fragment after hip dislocation. Three-dimensional tomography is very much useful before operation for difficult revisions of THR, reconstructions of acetabulum where one can get exact and clear picture, where there are ill-defined anatomy.

Q.24 What is utility of MRI?

Ans. Magnetic resonance imaging (MRI) is useful in transient osteoporosis, avascular necrosis, and benign and malignant tumours.

Q.25 What is the common stress fracture around hip?

Ans. Athelets can have stress fracture of femoral neck, pubic rami. Patients with osteomalacia can have bilateral stress fractures at subtrochanteric region.

Q.26 How do you assess bilateral external rotation deformity?

Ans. This can be done after putting both hips in 90° flexion and then can be assessed (Kothari's test).

Q.27 How do you assess bilateral adduction deformity?
Ans. The patient is put in supine position, vertical midline is drawn and a line perpendicular to it is drawn and a line is drawn joining both anterior superior iliac spines (ASIS). If there is deformity, then two lines are not parallel and accordingly adduction is measured.

Q.28 What is the method to measure rotation?
Ans. By two ways:
1. By assessing horizontal position of patella and upwards position of great toe, external or internal rotations are measured by rolling, or
2. This can be measured by flexing hip and knee 90° and outward rotation will indicate degree of internal rotation and inward rotation will indicate degree of external rotation.

Q.29 What is the position of ASIS in adduction and abduction deformity?
Ans. ASIS goes down in abduction deformity and is raised up in adduction deformity.

Q.30 Which is better informative test when both hips are affected?
Ans. Nelaton's line, which is drawn from ASIS to ischial tuberosity, touches normally tip of greater trochanter; but if both hips are affected, then both hips are above Nelaton's line, indicating proximal shifting of both trochanters.

Q.31 What is Bryant's triangle?
Ans. A circular line is drawn around at the level of ASIS joining both ASIS and a line is drawn from ASIS to tip of trochanter and a perpendicular line is drawn from tip to horizontal circular line and the length of this perpendicular line is measured and an inference is drawn about shifting of trochanter if there is unilateral affection such as posterior dislocation of hip, fracture neck of femur, excision arthroplasty of hip, Perthes' disease, coxa vara.
This test is not useful in bilateral affection.

Q.32 What are the causes of broadening of greater trochanter?
Ans. Healed or healing inter-trochanteric fracture, congenital coxa vara, Perthes' disease, tumour of greater trochanter, avascular necrosis (AVN) of head of femur, osteomyelitis of trochanter, etc.

Q.33 Which are the conditions when greater trochanter is close or away from ASIS?
Ans. Close—posterior dislocation.
Away—where there is increased external rotation such as anterior dislocation of hip, fracture neck of femur.

Q.34 Do you get some information about length in abduction deformity?
Ans. There is apparent lengthening in abduction deformity, when length is measured from umbilicus to tip of medial malleolus. If the difference of apparent

length and true length is taken, then apparent shortening is less than true shortening. Apparent length gives idea about compensation by making the pelvis oblique.

Q.35 How do you make the pelvis square?
Ans. One has to make the affected limb in abduction position to bring up lowered ASIS so as to bring both ASIS at same level and more adduction of affected limb to bring ASIS to lower level, raised ASIS on that side, and make the pelvis square.

Q.36 Is there any compensation spine in hip deformities? If so, what?
Ans. Yes, there is compensatory scoliosis of spine in abduction deformity.

Q.37 How much is abduction or adduction possible in both deformities respectively?
Ans. There is no further abduction possible in case of abduction deformity of hip and there is no further adduction possible in adduction of hip.

Q.38 How movements are assessed in the cases of hip deformities?
Ans. After squaring pelvis further abduction or adduction is done and likewise movements are assessed. Free abduction or adduction is taken into account without moving pelvis.

Q.39 How abduction or adduction deformity is calculated?
Ans. Both ASIS are joined by a line and then limb is moved either by abduction or adduction to square pelvis and the angle through which the affected ASIS is moved is measured and that is angle of deformity.

By Kothari's method, the angle is measured without squaring pelvis without any discomfort to patient, vertical midline is drawn and perpendicular lines are drawn to this midline and the angles are measured. Which give ideas of pelvic tilt.

Q.40 How do you measure lengths of both limbs?
Ans. One has to put normal limb in same deformity as affected limb and the lengths are measured.

Q.41 What are fallacies of squaring of pelvis?
Ans. Sometimes ASIS is removed for bone graft, maldeveloped pelvis, unreduced dislocations, malunited fractures of ilium, etc.

Q.42 What are reasons for true shortening?
Ans. Supratrochanteric—coxa vara, fracture neck of femur, Perthes' disease, absorption of neck, dislocation of hip, after girdlestone operation.

Infratrochanteric—congnital fracture shaft of femur, subtrochanteric fracture, , growth disturbances such as epiphyseal trauma.

Q.43 What causes lengthening of limb?
Ans. Supratrochanteric—coxa vagal, coax magna, and 5% cases of osteomyelitis (?may be due to vascular congestion).

Q.44 How much is extension possible in fixed flexion deformity?
Ans.
- Extension is not possible in flexion deformity.
- Extension is first movement to be lost in hip disease especially infective arthritis.

Q.45 Who described fixed flexion deformity?
Ans. By Sir Hugh Owen Thomas in 1876.

Q.46 Where is pathology when hip is not affected in flexion deformity?
Ans. There might be pathology either in pelvis or spine.

Q.47 How do you test fixed flexion deformity when knee is also flexion deformity?
Ans. Patient is asked to lie on edge of coach putting both knees dangling down and then fixed flexion is measured by Thomas test.

Q.48 What are difficulties in performing Thomas test?
Ans. Cannot be done in painful hips, obese patients, ankylosed knees and bilateral affected hips.

Q.49 When do you get false-positive Thomas test?
Ans. In cases of polio, scoliosis, exaggerated lordosis due to pregnancy spondylolisthesis, postural abnormalities, etc.

Q.50 How the range of movements presented when there are deformities of hip present?
Ans. When there is fixed adduction deformity—fixed addition + free adduction
When there is fixed abduction deformity—fixed abduction + free abduction
   When there is fixed flexion deformity, then fixed flexion + free flexion (For Ortolani's and Barlow's test, please see Chapter-13 Congenital Disorders).

17
CHAPTER

Tubercular Infection of Hip Joint

Q.1 What are common sites of focus in TB hip?
Ans. They are in order of preference—acetabular roof, head of femur, neck of femur and trochanter.

Q.2 What is type of tuberculosis of TB hip?
Ans. It is secondary to any primary lesion somewhere else such as lungs or glands and spread to hip by blood stream; usually, it starts as synovial lesion.

Q.3 What are stages of TB hip?
Ans.
- Stage I—tubercular synovitis
- Stage II—early arthritis
- Stage III—advanced arthritis
- Stage IV—advanced aortitis with subluxation or dislocation of hip.

Q.4 What are points favouring your diagnosis of TB hip?
Ans. TB hip is the disease of first three decades, slow and gradual onset, prolonged history, history of loss of weight and appetite, pain in hip may be referred to knee and there may be night cries, limp, tenderness at femoral triangle, typical deformities as per stage, wasting of muscle and apparent shortening as per the stage.

Q.5 What are means for confirmation of diagnosis of TB hip?
Ans.
Investigations:
- Blood examination—very high ESR, low haemoglobin, raised count of WBC, especially lymphocytes (lymphocytosis).
- ELISA test—for specific anti-tubercular proteins
- Radiologically—as per stages the changes are seen and assessed.
   Initially, there may be osteoporosis, diminished joint space, eroded articular surface, and destruction of head and neck in later stage.
   Even subluxation of dislocation (pathological) and wandering acetabulum is seen in very late stage.

Q.6 What are early signs of TB hip?

Ans. In the stage of synovitis, there may be abduction external rotation deformity and flexion to have maximum containment and joint space to have infective debris and pus, if any.

Q.7 What can be differential diagnosis of early stage deformity of TB hip?

Ans. Perthes' disease, iliopsoas spasm, slipped capital femoral epiphysis, low-grade septic arthritis, rheumatoid arthritis, traumatic synovitis.

Q.8 What is normal course of TB hip, if untreated?

Ans. If untreated, there can be stable fibrous ankylosis, may be in good functional position or unfunctional position.

Q.9 What is aim of treatment?

Ans. To get mobile joint when presented at early stage of disease. But if presented at later stage, then it should be sound stable ankylosis in functional position so as to get stable and painless hip.

Q.10 What is differential diagnosis of arthritic stage?

Ans. Monoarticular rheumatoid arthritis, Perthes' disease, old healed septic arthritis.

Q.11 What are differentiating points?

Ans.
- Monoarticular rheumatoid—usually there is flexion, abduction and external rotation deformity
- Perthes' disease—adduction and external rotation
- In septic arthtritis—all movements are painful and restricted.

Q.12 What is treatment of TB hip?

Ans. Skin traction to correct deformity—Multiple-drug therapy for at least 9 months—first-4-drug therapy is started for 2 months, then shifted to two or three-drug therapy for remaining period.

Rest to part by hip spica—Rehabilitation by gentle exercises and gradual weight bearing is started from partial (after 12 weeks) to full weight bearing within few months.

Q.13 Why extra-articular arthrodesis is done?

Ans. Before introduction of anti-tubercular drug therapy it was thought dangerous to open joint because of dissemination of disease, so arthrodesis was done without opening joint.

Q.14 Does traction help in TB hip?

Ans. If it is early stage, then it relieves spasm and tries to correct deformity, if any, articular surfaces are kept apart thus minimising destruction and minimising risk of migration or dislocation and thus preventing wandering acetabulum.

Q.15 How do you treat it in advanced stage?
Ans. If there is more destruction, then the aim is for arthrodesis in functional position such as 5–10° external rotation, flexion up to 30° as per age, and 15° abduction.

Q.16 What are indications of surgery in TB hip?
Ans.
- When response to conservative treatment fails.
- When outcome of conservative treatment is not favourable.

Q.17 What operations can be done for TB hip?
Ans.
- Synovectomy and debridement (removal) of loose bodies, debris, pannus, loose articular cartilage and careful curettage of tubercular lesion of bone if any, of joint—can be done at synovial stage, no response to treatment or no confirmation of diagnosis.
- When the disease has ended with fibrous ankylosis with some deformity, then upper femoral corrective osteotomy for flexion and adduction displacement of femur and correction for fibrous ankylosis.
- If there is unsound ankylosis in nonfunctional position, then arthrodesis is the only answer either extra-articular or intra-articular and deformity is corrected if any ischiofemoral, iliofemoral, etc.
- Girdlestone excision arthroplasty, if movements are to be aimed followed by stabilising osteotomy such as bachelor's osteotomy.
- THR in totally healed cases.

Q.18 What are advantages and disadvantages of arthrodesis?
Ans. Usually, it is done in children, usually extra-articular to avoid growth disturbances —good stable painless hip and children learn to compromise with position of hip, there are compensatory adjustment at spine in children.
Disadvantages—loss of all movements, cannot squat or sit cross-legged.

Q.19 What are advantages and disadvantages of Girdlestone operation?
Ans. Advantage—painless mobile hip, useful in adults
Disadvantages—unstable hip, if acetabulum is affected pain is not relieved completely, shortening.

Q.20 Who described excision arthroplasty operation and when?
Ans. Girdlestone described in 1950 an excision of femoral head, neck, proximal part of trochanter, and rim of acetabulum, etc.

Q.21 What is postoperative management after Girdlestone operation?
Ans. Limb is kept in abduction of 30°–50° and skeletal tibial traction is applied on Bohler's spint for 6 weeks, with 10–15 kg weight so as to get gap between excised head part and acetabulum, filled with fibrous tissue and minimising unstability. And to form pseudoarthrosis and followed by stabilising osteotomy.

Q.22 When can one do THR in TB hip?

Ans. Usually after 10 years and when the disease is quiescent and there are no evidences of tuberculosis. But there is no definite answer to this.

Q.23 Is there any difference between TB hip of child and adult?

Ans. Yes, in adults due to bizarre treatment now and then, there is no typical picture of tuberculosis of hip such as deformity, etc. So one can aim for mobile hip in adult by excision arthroplasty or so. The movements are not restricted as they get restricted in children and there is less osteoporosis.

18 CHAPTER

Slipped Capital Femoral Epiphysis

Q.1 What is slipped capital femoral epiphysis?
Ans. Slipped capital femoral epiphysis (SCFE) is usual posterior displacement or slipping of proximal femoral epiphysis on the femoral neck.

Q.2 What are predisposing factors?
Ans. Obese males (2–3 times more than females of ages between 8 and 16 years), rarely trauma, inflammation, endocrine and renal disorders, nutritional deficiencies, history of irradiation therapy. Still exact cause is unknown.

The children are overweight, there is excessive femoral retroversion and thus mechanical factor plays significant role to make prone to slipping and unstable.

Q.3 What is clinical picture of SCFE?
Ans. The onset may be acute or insidious over months, usual symptoms are pain in the groin, along medial side of thigh, or knee, limitations of hip movements, especially internal rotation; in chronic cases, there may be shortening and external rotation.

Q.4 What is classification of SCFE?
Ans. Acute—sudden onset for 2 weeks or less
Chronic—symptoms for more than 2 weeks and X-ray shows callus formation and signs of remodelling
Acute-cum-chronic—symptoms present more than 1 month with sudden exacerbation of pain.
Preslip—X-ray showing irregularity, widening and fuzziness of physics

Another way of classification:
Stable—where child can bear weight with or without crutches
Unstable—severe pain makes child to bear weight even with crutches.

Based on displacement:
Mild—one third or less of femoral head slipping,
Moderate—one third to one half of femoral diameter epiphysis has slipped
Severe—more than one half of femoral diameter, the epiphysis has slipped.

Q.5 What is effective treatment?

Ans. *Principle of treatment*—stabilisation of slipping process and premature closure of physis.
- *For stable slips*—6-7 mm cannulated screw (partially or fully threaded) is inserted percutaneous *in situ*, into centre of epiphysis under image intensifier television (IITV) and insertion of screw starts anterior to neck of femur, slip, is posterior. In severe slip the screw is passed more anteriorly.
- *Unstable slips*—preoperative traction (skin or skeletal) for reduction of slip is used for 2-3 weeks and many times there is spontaneous reduction occurs under anaesthesia and screw is inserted under IITV in desired position. Open reduction is very rarely required.

Q.6 What are other methods of treatment of SCFE?

Ans. Some form of reconstructive surgery has to be done in moderately and severely displaced epiphysis. Different osteotomies are advised and done to restore normal relationship of femoral head and neck to delay degenerative joint disease. The Indications of osteotomy are problems with gait, sitting, and cosmetic appearance one year after stabilizing operations, malunion of chronic slip in poor position. Femoral osteotomy is done for correction of deformity but osteonecrosis is reported in 2-100% of patients. Compensatory osteotomy is safer as it is distal to major blood supply in the posterior retinaculum and so chances of osteonecrosis are minimum but it causes shortening of the femoral neck to some extent.

Intertrochanteric or subtrochanteric osteotomies can provide good reorientation of capital physis with minimum risk of osteonecrosis.

There are few osteotomies such as osteotomy through neck near epiphysis, through base of neck, through trochanteric region are advised.

Q.7 What are complications after treatment?

Ans. Most serious is osteonecrosis, which is rare in untreated slips and infrequent in stable slips after fixing with pins *in situ*. It is observed that osteonecrosis occurs in 47% cases in unstable slips which are not reduced before fixation. Reduction with force should not be attempted otherwise more chances of osteonecrosis.

Chondrolysis—less frequent complications (3-7%)

Further slipping—in spite of pinning occurs in slips with associated with some endocrinopathies, unstable slips.

CHAPTER 19

Legg-Calvé-Perthes Disease

Q.1 What is Legg-Calvé-Perthes (LCP) disease?
Ans. Legg-Calvé-Perthes disease is idiopathic avascular necrosis of femoral head, occurring in children.

Q.2 Which age group is affected by LCP disease?
Ans. The most common age is 5–9 years, but it is seen in 18 months old child and 18 years old adolescent also.

Q.3 Why this disease has complex name?
Ans. As it was discovered by Arthur Legg of Boston, Jacques Calvé of France and George Perthes of Germany in 1909 while studying children for tuberculosis found mild symptoms without tuberculosis of hip which was found out with newly invented X-ray machine. Actually Dr Waldenstrom of Sweden found and described pervious to theses authors but he labeled as mild tuberculosis.

Q.4 What is etiology of LCP disease?
Ans. No particular cause is assigned so far but there are theories—Theory of thrombolysis— where the children are deficient in some protein S or C or thrombolysin and changes in femoral head may be due to arterial or venous infarction, second one is more likely.

Q.5 How do you diagnose this LCP disease?
Ans. *Clinically*—child has limping, occasional pain either in hip or knee, no history of injury, insidious onset, on examination there is mild limp with decreased range of movements of affected hip especially internal rotation.

Radiologically—Anteroposterior (AP) and lateral X-rays are taken which reveal increase in density of femoral head. X-ray may be repeated if initial X-ray is negative after a month. Bone scan or MRI may clinch to early diagnosis

Q.6 How does the progress of disease occur?
Ans. There are four stages of this disease:
- Initial stage—in which femoral head is dense.
- Fragmentation stage—where femoral head is soft and deformed.
- Healing stage—where new bone grows into femoral head
- Residual stage—healed femoral head which is deformed.

Clinically at early stage, there is intermittent synovitis with limp and pain and irritability of hip. The symptoms increase with activity and relief with rest. In the stage of fragmentation, there is more loss of movements of hip, especially internal rotation and abduction after year or so there is improvement of symptoms and after 2 years the patient is normal with some complaints such as mild limp, pain and some decrease in movements.

Q.7 What are prognostic signs?

Ans. The older the child the worst is outcome at onset. So, if the onset is before 6 years, then outcome is better than older age group such as after 9 years where there is severity of symptoms with deformed head not responding to treatment. Early detection of LCPD is essential to get a good end result with a spherical head.

Q.8 How do you classify severity of disease?

Ans. Group A—no change in lateral pillar (lateral third of femoral head) and these do well even without any active treatment.

Group B—head with partial collapse (upto 50%) of lateral buttress of femoral head and have intermediate prognosis.

Group C—head has collapse more than 50% of lateral pillar and do not respond well to treatment.

Q.9 What is form of early treatment?

Ans.
- Observation of child
- Restriction of vigorous sports and activities
- Complete bed rest.

If not still relieved, then use of non-weight-bearing devices such as crutch walking or use of weight-relieving caliper.

Q.10 What is classification of LCP disease?

Ans. There are several different classifications used to determine severity of disease and prognosis.

The *Catteral Classification* specifies four different groups to define radiographic appearance during the period of greatest bone loss.

The *Salter-Thomson Classification* simplifies the Catteral Classifications by reducing them down to two groups: Group A (Catteral I, II) which shows that less than 50% of the ball is involved, and Group B (Catteral III, IV) where more than 50% of the ball is involved. Both classifications share the view that if less than 50% of the ball is involved, the prognosis is good, while more than 50% involvement indicates a potentially poor prognosis.

The *Herring Classification* studies the integrity of the lateral pillar of the ball. In the Lateral Pillar Group A, there is no loss of height in the lateral 1/3 of the head and little density change. In Lateral Pillar Group B, there is lucency and loss of height of less than 50% of the lateral height. Sometimes, the ball is beginning to extrude the socket. In Lateral Pillar Group C, there is more than 50% loss of lateral height.

Q.11 What is surgical treatment of LCP disease?

Ans. *Surgical Treatment*

Tenotomy: A "Tenotomy" is a surgery that is performed to release an atrophied muscle that has shortened due to limping. Once released, a cast is applied allowing the muscle to regrow to a more natural length. Cast time is about 6–8 weeks.

Osteotomy: There are different types of "osteotomies" (cutting the bone to reposition it) and, depending on the need they are performed at different stages of the disease. At times with the softening of the ball, there is the possibility of the ball slipping out of the socket. To protect it, a femoral varus osteotomy, with or without rotation partially redirects the ball into the socket.

Another approach to surgically treating Legg-Calve-Perthes is to do an osteotomy above the hip socket. This allows the surgeon to reposition the hip socket in such a way that the femoral head will have less tendency to become deformed. The shelf arthroplasty gives added coverage of the ball from the top lip of the socket. Both the innominate and the shelf arthroplasty help in reshaping.

Core decompression: This simple procedure is used in mild to moderate cases. A hole is created in the bone and a part of the bone is removed from the hip area. The use of crutches is necessary for 6 weeks after the procedure to avoid fracturing the bone.

The transphyseal neck to head femoral drilling. The cases of ischemic disease of the growing hip (IDGH) stage II and III, were transphyseal neck-head drilling have been used, did not progressed to LCPD, and the preliminary study of the epidemiological data seemed to show a decrease on the incidence of the illness on our population. Those facts point to a preventive effect of this intervention on the onset of LCPD. We have begun now a prospective double blind study to confirm those results.

Bone grafting: The dead bone is removed and a bone graft is put in its place. The bone graft is taken from the patient or from a bone bank. Crutches and/or walkers will need to be used for up to a year to help the healing process.

Vascularized bone grafting: Similar to above procedure, the dead bone is removed and a bone graft is put in its place. The difference is that in vascularized bone grafting the bone graft comes with its own blood vessels. The body then does not have to create a fresh blood supply.

Femoral head resurfacing: A metal head is placed over the original femoral head to slow the progression of the disease. Over time, a complete femoral head replacement will need to be performed.

Femoral head replacement: The femoral head is replaced and a stem is placed inside the femoral bone.

Total hip replacement: Once the disease has progressed to the point, the hip socket is affected, a total hip replacement may be necessary. Hip replacements are usually successful. The downside is that with today's technology, a total hip replacement may not last as long as the life of the patient. That is why surgeons will wait to perform the operation until it is absolutely necessary.

CHAPTER 20

Fracture Neck of Femur

Q.1 What are types of fracture neck of femur?
Ans.
- Undisplced/impacted
- Displaced.

Q.2 How do you diagnose impacted fracture neck of femur?
Ans.
- Groin pain which may be referred to knee
- Antalgic gait
- Limited and painful hip movements.

Q.3 What are signs and symptoms of displaced fracture neck of femur?
Ans.
- Minimal shortening,
- Generalised pain with externally rotated thigh and abduction.

Q.4 How do you classify fracture neck of femur?
Ans.
- Intracapsular—subcapital and transcervical
- Extracapsular—intertrochanteric and subtrochanteric.

Q.5 How do you diagnose old fracture neck of femur?
Ans.
- Tender midinguinal point (anteriorly)
- Positive telescopic test due to absorption of neck
- Crepitus may be present
- Absence of transmitted movements at neck but present at trochanter.

Q.6 How do you do telescopic test?
Ans. Patient is on hard bed (preferably), pelvis is fixed with one hand, hip and knee are flexed at 90° and with another hand with knee to and fro movements are done and telescopic movements are felt by hand which is at trochanter and fixing pelvis. This test has to be experienced by one self and felt by every body. Other no proper appreciation.

Q.7 What is common deformity after fracture neck off femur?

Ans. Adduction due to weight-bearing when walking is attempted.

Q.8 How do differentiate old fracture neck of femur and trochanter fracture?

Ans. In fracture neck of femur-lower age group, trivial injury, less ecchymosis and tender midinguinal region, pain at this point after bitrochanteric compression test, minimal shortening, no external rotation in impacted fracture of neck of femur and some external rotation in displaced fractures, telescopic test positive (in old case), vascular sign of Narath is positive in old cases due to absorption of neck, normal trochanter, less supratrochanteric shortening, high percentage of nonunion (10–30%) avascular necrosis quite common (15–30%).

In old trochanteric fracture, elderly age group due to osteoporosis, lateral ecchymosis, lateral part tender, marked external rotation, marked shortening, absent transmitted movements, negative or false positive.

Telescopic test (after nonunion but with marked shortening), negative.

Narath's vascular sign—pain at trochanter after bitrochanteric compression test, uncommon nonunion (1%), most common malunion (coxa vara) more supratrochanteric shortening, (with severe trauma this fracture may occur in young adults), broad and thickened greater trochanter very rare avascular necrosis (basal fractures).

Q.9 How will you treat impacted or undisplaced fracture neck of femur?

Ans. There is always risk of displacement of fracture as there is almost no pain or less pain patient tries to bear weight and the fracture gets displaced. So, it is better to treat these fractures also by surgery such as 3-4 parallel cannulated lag screws. This can be done percutaneously with help of IITV.

Q.10 What are different types of treatment available for fresh fracture neck of femur?

Ans. In children (adolescents)—multiple pinning.

In adults—Dynamic hip screw is most preferred because of sliding effect of the implant.

In older days, Smith Peterson nailing was done most commonly.

All operations are aimed to get osteosynthesis and early prompt reduction either closed or open with internal fixation is most recommended.

In elderly patients hemiarthroplasty, bipolar arthroplasty or total arthroplasty is done primarily, depending upon condition of patient, at least after age (chronological or biological) of 60 years. Usually, attempt of osteosynthesis is done but fails due to many reasons mainly due to osteoporosis. And patient may not stand for two major operations.

Early reduction and holding in reduced position may reduce chances of avascular necrosis and nonunion.

Q.11 How do you reduce fracture neck of femur?

Ans. *Leadbetter's method*—pelvis is stabilised, hip and knee are flexed, held up for some time to disengage the fragments, then abduction of hip is done with internal rotation with extension of hip. Ultimately, the limb is kept in 10-15° of internal rotation and proper traction is applied with help of traction device of orthopaedic table.

Q.12 What are bony complications even after good internal fixation and for displaced fracture neck of femur?

Ans.
- Nonunions: 10-30%
- Avascular necrosis 15-35% (it is more in adoscents)
- Late segmental collapse.

Q.13 When absorption of neck appears?

Ans. By at least third week.

Q.14 What are major bony complications after hemiarthroplasty?

Ans.
- Hip pain due to implant loosening, and erosion of acetabulum
- Dislocation of implanted hip
- Femoral shaft fracture may be during reduction of metallic head (may be spiral fracture)
- Heterotopic ossification
- Painful movements or stiffness of hip may be due to wrong selection of size of implant or expansion of metallic head due to heat following walking.

Q.15 What is avascular necrosis?

Ans. There is actual death of bone in femoral head following to ischemia.

Q.16 What is late segmental collapse?

Ans. This is collapse of subchondral bone and articular cartilage over lying necrotic bone results in congruency of joint leading to degenerative arthritis and pain.

Q.17 What you get avascular necrosis in each and every patient of fracture neck of femur?

Ans. No, with proper, early good anatomical reduction and internal fixation bone which has got avascular necrosis many times get repaired and revascularised.

Q.18 Name the surgeon who invented first implant for fracture neck of femur.

Ans. Von Langenback.

Q.19 Do you get avascular necrosis even after good fixation and when?

Ans. Yes, sometimes even after union of fracture also one can get avascular necrosis as late as after 2 years of operation.

Q.20 What is method to treat ipsilateral femoral neck fracture and femoral shaft fracture?

Ans. Anatomic reduction of femoral neck fracture and with stable internal fixation and femoral shaft is fixed with plate and screw or long gamma nails can give better result which can fix neck and shaft also.

Q.21 What is Garden's index?

Ans. Compression trabeculae forms an angle of 160° in AP and 180° in lateral view. The ratio is known as Garden's index which gives idea of anatomic reduction for femoral neck fractures.

Q.22 Is there any role of anteversion, retroversion in good reduction?

Ans. If retroversion is not rectified by doing internal rotation of limb during operation immediately after reduction, then there will not be proper fixation and implant may be out.

Q.23 Why prosthetic replacement is done in old patients?

Ans. In osteoporotic bones implant hold may be poor and due to that implant may back out when attempted for osteosynthesis. After failure of this old patients may not withstand for second operation, and early mobilisation can be done with prosthetic replacement. There are great chances of avascular necrosis (AVN) and nonunion in old patients.

Q.24 When do you do hemiarthroplasty? Which and why?

Ans. Absolute indications are, old fractures with or without AVN, old age, no good anatomic reduction, bony disease in the head of femur with fracture.

Relative indications—osteoporosis, poor general conditions of patient, bed-ridden patient, fracture with dislocation.

Austin Moore prosthesis is done when good calcar is present. Thomson's prosthesis is used when calcar is not present.

Q.25 What is Ward's triangle or Babcock's triangle?

Ans. Ward's triangle—lateral to principle compression and below tension trabeculae. This is avoided during fixation.

Babcock's—inferior sector of head where fixation is poor.

Q.26 Which reduction is better for fixation?

Ans. Valgus reduction and alignment is preferred as it controls better collapse and overcome bending by shear.

Q.27 Which is better approach for hemiarthroplasty?

Ans. This is posterior hip approach used in America for first time, so it is named southern America or Philadelphia approach.

Q.28 Which is better arthroplasty bipolar or Austin Moore's Prosthesis?

Ans. Bipolar is better one as there is better 3 point fixation due to long stem and straight implant less friction and impact forces between implant and articular cartilage can be easily converted into total hip replacement (THR).

Q.29 What are the complications of bipolar?

Ans. Loosening, acetabular wear and tear, pain, and increased incidence of dislocation.

Q.30 What are advantages of bipolar?

Ans. Removes all shear forces, less incidence of protrusio acetabula, and easily convertible to THR.

Q.31 What are fixation points of prosthesis?

Ans. There are three points fixation:
1. Medial cortex of shaft by stem of implant
2. Head
3. Trochanter

Q.32 What are indications of THR after femoral neck fractures?

Ans. Displaced femoral neck fractures in elderly patients above age of 60 with diseases in hip and acetabulum such rheumatoid arthritis, osteoarthritis, Paget's disease, or pathological fracture when acetabulum is affected.

Q.33 Who invented bipolar?

Ans. James Batman.

Q.34 What is McMurray's osteotomy?

Ans. It is an oblique (45°) subtrochanteric osteotomy done (in direction of lower end of acetabulum) from below upward, inside to outside, with medial displacement of distal fragment with abduction of limb to compensate the length as there is shortening after this osteotomy.

This was described by McMurray for primary osteoarthritis of hip to relieve pain. Due to medial displacement of distal fragment, there is change in weight-bearing axis and forces on the femoral neck fracture are reduced which in turn gives good union. The main purpose is change of axis of weight bearing and when osteotomy site gets united patient may walk comfortably.

Q.35 What is postoperative regime after McMurray's osteotomy?

Ans. In young adults, full hip spica for 6 weeks to start in full abduction and the hip spica is changed by keeping the limb into less abduction (or adduction as much as possible).

In elderly people, it is better to use some kind of internal fixation such as Van Wright plate, etc. to avoid stiffness which is common after hip spica, so hip spica is not applied.

Q.36 What are indications of McMurray's osteotomy?
Ans. Nonunion of neck of femur, osteoarthritis of hip when THR cannot be done.

Q.37 What are disadvantages of this operation?
Ans. Shortening, not easy to convert to THR, if needed, cannot sit cross-legged.

Q.38 Who was the first to do prosthesis?
Ans. Heygroove (1920) used ivory endoprosthesis.

Q.39 What is evolution of prosthesis?
Ans.
- Heygroove (1920)—ivory
- Judet (1948)—Acrylic
- Moore and Bohlman (1940)—metallic prosthesis
- Thomson (1954)
- Austin Moore (1955)
- Bipolar-Batmann (1978).

Q.40 What is postoperative management with dynamic hip screw?
Ans. Non-weight-bearing exercises to be started immediately second day such as sitting in bed mobilisation of hip and knee.
- Crutch walking—first week (non-weight-bearing)
- Partial weight bearing—6th week
- Total weight bearing—8 weeks
- In elderly people—one has to more cautious as there is osteoporosis and implant may back out.

Q.41 How do you manage postoperatively prosthesis cases (hemiarthroplasty)?
Ans. Patient can be made to stand as soon as possible and when patient is stable and when ambulation is tolerated a pillow between thighs is preferable.

Q.42 What is blood supply of head of femur?
Ans. Medial circumflex femoral artery and lateral circumflex femoral artery are main blood suppliers of head, by their medial, posterior and anterior ascending branches all these are branches of Profundus artery (4/5 head)
Arteries of ligamentum teres (medial epiphyseal arteries of Trueta) (1/5 head) but this artery is absent in 20–30% people.

Q.43 How Garden has classified femoral neck fractures?
Ans.
- Incomplete
- Complete impacted
- Partially displaced
- Completely displaced.

Q.44 What is Pauwel's classification?
Ans. Based on angle of fracture with imaginary horizontal line:
- 30°—subcapital
- 50°—transcervical
- 70° basal—unites early and in better way

This is better for old age group.

Q.45 What is classification in children?
Ans. Epiphysis is present, so this is taken into account:
- Transepiphyseal
- Transcervical
- Cervicotrochanteric
- Intertrochanteric.

Q.46 What is angle of neck of femur?
Ans. It is 130° to 135° in males and it is 120° to 125° in females. And approximately 140° to 150° in children.

Q.47 What are problems while doing THR?
Ans. There are 21% medical complications in osteoarthritis (OA) including dislocations of hip, but less than when THR done for OA of hip.

Usually, fracture of femur (old) is given as long case and you should be prepared very well for proper examination, diagnosis, and treatment including recent ones. You should be very well in your basic signs.

CHAPTER 21

Intertrochanteric Fracture

Q.1 What is a fracture of trochanter?
Ans. An intertrochanteric fracture is extracapsular fracture of neck of femur, which occurs along a line between greater and lesser trochanters with variable comminution.

Q.2 How do you classify trochanteric fractures?
Ans.
- Intertrochanteric fracture—47%
- Subtrochanteric fractures—23%
- Femoral neck fractures—37%.

Q.3 What are the classifications of trochanteric fracture?
Ans.
- Boyd and Griffins
- Tronzo
- Evans
- AO classification.

Q.4 What is subtrochanteric fracture?
Ans. A subtrochanteric fracture is fracture occurring between lesser trochanter and point 5 cm distal to lesser trochanter.

Q.5 What are the classifications of subtrochanteric fracture?
Ans. Based on distance at or below lesser trochanter (Fielding)—the more distal fracture the more are complications.

Based on number of major fragments and location and shape of fracture line (Seinsheimer) more comminuted fracture result in more complications.
Another way—stable, where bone to bone contact is established in the medial and posterior cortices, unstable—it is not possible to have medial cortex apposition due to more comminution and obliquity of fracture.

Q.6 What are methods to treat intertrochanteric fractures?
Ans. *Conservative*
- By simple skin traction
- By Hamilton Russel traction
- By tibial traction.

Operative
- By simple Smith Peterson nail and plate
- By Jewetts nail plate
- By modified Talwalkar's nail and plate
- By dynamic hip screw
- By Enders nails
- By right angled dynamic hip screw
- By external fixators.

Q.7 Which is the best method to treat these fractures?
Ans. When patients are not suitable for surgery then treatment by conservative tibial traction for at least 2 to 3 months.

When patients with fit for surgery then dynamic hip screw has better hold and due to its sliding property collapse of fracture is controlled in better way without protrusion of implant.

So, no one implant is most ideal one.

Q.8 How do you reduce trochanteric fracture on table?
Ans. First patient is taken on fracture table, pelvis is stabilised by an assistant, then affected hip is flexed, kept in flexion for some time and then by giving gentle traction limb is extended and fixed on fracture table. Suitable traction is given with adjustment of fracture table, finally limb is kept in internal rotation. When lesser trochanter is displaced to good extend, when there is a more comminution then the limb has to keep in external rotation to close fracture gap.

Q.9 What are the features of instability?
Ans. Severe posteromedial comminution:
- Mark shortening
- Varus of neck shaft angles
- Increased retroversion.

Q.10 What are the complication of trochanteric fractures?
Ans. Malunion—most common as there is good amount of osteoporosis in elderly people and there is a collapse.
Marked shortening
Nonunion—very uncommon—1%
Avascular necrosis—less than 0.8%.

Q.11 What are the postoperative complications of implant fixation in trochanteric fractures?
Ans.
- Infection
- Breaking of nail at nail plate junction
- Protrusion of implant or cutting of the bone by implant
- Shortening.

Intertrochanteric Fracture

Q.12 How do you measured length of DHS screw?
Ans. The screw should be within 1.5 cm of subcontrol level of head of femur.

Q.13 Where do you place guidewire?
Ans. The ideal placement of guidewire is parallel to calcar, midline of the head of the femur (preferably in lower quadrant) as trabeculae of calcar are stronger than any-where. The placement of the nail in superior quadrant of the head is of potential danger.

Q.14 What is Sarmiento's operation?
Ans. It is an oblique osteotomy at 45° followed by medialization.

Q.15 What is Dimon and Hugston operation?
Ans. A transverse osteotomy of shaft is done and distal portion is medialised. This Hugston procedure is good for unstable intertrochanteric fracture with comminution of calcar, posterior arch and posterior arch along with shaft. So, restoration is necessary for this.

Q.16 What are the trochanteric prosthesis?
Ans. Leinbach's prosthesis is specially designed for trochanteric fractures.

Q.17 What are the indications for doing trochanteric prosthesis?
Ans.
- Severe osteoporosis
- Severe comminution
- Life with low activity (old age and debility)
- When proximal fixation cannot be done.

Q.18 How do you treat malunited trochanteric fractures?
Ans. There is external rotation with marked shortening, so subtrochanteric osteotomy has to be done and not attend to compensate of length is made.
    Adductor tenotomy may be done.
    With ring fixators now a days one can get good length and correction of deformity by doing corrective osteotomy and by gradual distraction (Ilizarov method).

Q.19 What is a calcar?
Ans. A dense pattern of trabeculae, which are stronger running a long inferior border of neck of femur and extending into the shaft along lesser trochanter is a calcar, if implant is put along the calcar then its stabilises in better way.

Q.20 How do you assess the strength of fracture implant combination?
Ans. It depends upon degree of osteoporosis, fragment geometry, proper reduction, design of implant and placement of the implant.

CHAPTER 22

Total Hip Replacement

Q.1 What are the causes of arthritis?
Ans. *Noninflammatory:* This includes idiopathic osteoarthritis and post-traumatic degeneration of joint, congenital deformities and avascular necrosis.
Inflammatory: Rheumatoid arthritis, connective tissue disease leading to arthritis, lupus erythematous and psoriatic arthritis.

Q.2 How osteoarthritis is presented?
Ans. Pain, inability to sleep, limping, absence of active flexion, range of motion is reduced, and walking distance is also lessened (gradually). Constant pain in groin may be due to irritation of obturator nerve which runs directly to hip joint.

Q.3 How X-ray looks like in arthritis?
Ans. Narrowing of joint space, formation of osteophytes, and subchondral cysts.

Q.4 How osteophytes are formed?
Ans. Following degeneration of articular cartilage, stress on bone gets increased and to get more surface area for increased stress laying down of new bone takes place which is called osteophyte (Wolff's law).

Q.5 Describe mechanism of subchondral cysts?
Ans. Due to high stress, stress fractures occur and due to continued pressure. These fractures do not heal and cysts are formed. After removal of stress such by operation of THR or so cysts heal and are filled with bone.

Q.6 How do you treat osteoarthritis (OA) of hip without operation?
Ans. By using anti-inflammatory drugs, using cane in opposite hand to decrease reactive force on affected joint, and attempt to reduce weight (if overweight is there) may be tried for at least for 6 months.

Q.7 What are the operations done for OA of hip?
Ans. Femoral osteotomies, such as McCurray's test, etc. with concept of relieving subchondral venous engorgement, changing of weight-bearing axis, hip arthroscopic surface arthroplasty (has shown some benefits), excision arthroplasty, cup arthroplasty (in olden days) surf arthroplasty (new technique).

Q.8 What are the common approaches for hip surgery?

Ans. Most common are—posterior, direct lateral, anterolateral, and posterolateral are most commonly followed and are very popular.

Q.9 What are advantages and disadvantages?

Ans. *Posterior:* Easy to do, easy to see femur, and postoperative limp is uncommon. *Disadvantages:* Difficult to see complete acetabulum and postoperative increased incidences of dislocations.

Transtrochanteric advantages: Easy to do with more exposure but more incidences of trochanteris nonunions and limp.

Anterolateral advantages: Easy to do with good exposure and low incidences of dislocations but there is more incidences of limp and heterotopic bone formation.

Q.10 What is modern femoral cement technique?

Ans. This includes plugging of distal femur, washing and drying of canal use of cement gun to fill canal from distal to proximal and there should be pressure on cement. Even some surgeons recommend vacuum mixing or centrifugation to lessen porosity of cement.

Q.11 Why one should use cementless stems?

Ans. By using cementless one gets advantage creating biologic interface for fixation. As cement is non-biologic interface, which reacts to stresses and strength but there can be early loosening of previous stable femoral stem.

Q.12 What is size of pores to have bone in growth?

Ans. Many agree that pore size should be between 100–450 microns. So that there can be 30–40% porous in growth of well fixed fully porous coated femoral stem.

Q.13 What is good design of cement less acetabular component?

Ans. Acetabular component should be circular in shape, fully porous coated and placed in press fit (tight) fashion. Screw fixation of component is doubtful.

Q.14 What sizes of head and liner are to be used?

Ans. If 26–28 mm head is used then there are less chances of dislocation than to small size of head where there is minimum friction and wear with at least 6 mm polyethylene in the socket.

Q.15 What is intraoperative vascular effect of cement in THR?

Ans. The cement is vasodilator and may cause sudden hypotension and may cause sudden death on the table, so the patient has to be well hydrated and with vasopressor drugs. There may be anaphylactic reaction also so anesthetist should be alarmed while passing cement especially in femoral stem.

Q.16 Which nerves are injured in THR? How?

Ans. The most common nerve involved in the injury is sciatic nerve (79%), then femoral nerve (13%) and most uncommon is obturator nerve. The causes of these injuries are unknown in 47% cases, due to traction in 20% cases, due to contusion in 18%, due to hematoma in 11%.

Q.17 What precautions one has to take while putting screws in acetabular component?

Ans. An area which is anterior to line drawn from anterior superior iliac spine to dividing acetabulum into two halves, should be avoided as important structures are lying deep to bony pelvis such as external iliac artery, and vein, and obturator nerve, vein and artery. The screw placed in this may cause injuries to these structures.

Q.18 What are the causes of intraoperative femoral fractures?

Ans. They are:
- Improper reaming of femoral canal
- Putting large component in the canal
- Attempts to pound the component down the canal too rapidly without allowing viscoelastic nature of bone to accept component
- Failure to appreciate preoperative deformities and narrowing of distal femoral canal.

Q.19 What is incidence of thrombophlebitis in untreated patients? How many lead to pulmonary embolism?

Ans. It is approx 50% and 0.1–0.2% cases may have pulmonary emboilism.

Q.20 How will you prevent?

Ans. By early mobilisation, compression stockings or elastocrepe bandages and use of anticoagulants such as warfarin, aspirin, heparin, low molecular heparin and dextran.

Q.21 How will you prevent dislocation after operation?

Ans. By avoiding excessive flexion, internal rotation, adduction and combinations of extensive extension, external rotation and adduction.

Q.22 What are common causative organisms of infection in THR?

Ans. Most common—*Staphylococcus aureus*, but *Staphylococcus epidermidis* common in prosthetic operations.

Q.23 How infection can be prevented or minimised?

Ans.
- Proper preoperative check and treatment for dental infection, or infection anywhere in the body
- Good and healthy skin
- Prophylactic antibiotics
- Reducing traffic in patient's room
- Laminar airflow within enclosed area
- Fast surgery, meticulous hemostasis, and proper wound care.
  Still potential infection may reveal even after one year of surgery.

Q.24 What is osteolysis?
Ans. Severe absorption of bone around prosthesis mediated by collagenases, prostaglandins and proteases.

Q.25 Describe long-term common complication.
Ans. Loosening which causes pain.

Q.26 What radiological signs of loose component?
Ans. X-ray reveals (a) migration of component, (b) fracture of cement, (c) 2 mm lucent line surrounding prothesis.

Q.27 What is cause of osteolysis?
Ans. Due to wear of polyethylene of cup there is debris of polyethylene which goes down to the femur, around edges of cup or through screws of cup.

Q.28 How can it be prevented?
Ans. By using proper size of head (26–28 mm), maximum polyethylene thickness (at least 6 mm), alternative bearing surface such ceramics or metal, and highly cross-linked polyethylene.

Q.29 What measures are taken to prevent hematogenous infection?
Ans. With preoperative antibiotics, proper care of dental infection if any and aggressive treatment for infection.

Q.30 What are the steps to prevent heterotopic bone formation in high-risk patients?
Ans. Minimum handling of tissues during operation, eliminating the debris of femoral canal after reaming, a single dose of 600 rads on 3–4th day after operation. Drug indomethacin can be used.

Q.31 What are general principles of treatment of infected THR?
Ans. Prolonged course of antibiotics and surgery.

Q.32 What is typical antibiotic regimen for treatment of infected THR?
Ans. The broad-spectrum antibiotic such as first generation cephalosporin—Cefazolin or methicillin or oxacillin, once after culture when organism is identified proper antibiotic should started. At least for 4–6 weeks.

Q.33 What are options are available for infected THR?
Ans. Two stage implantation, one stage implantation, resection arthroplasty, thorough debridement with retention of old implant, chronic suppressive antibiotics without any surgery, arthroscopic debridement, hip arthrodesis, and hip disarticulation.

Q.34 Which operation has better prospects?
Ans. Two stage reimplantation is better solution, which has given 92% success rate.

Q.35 What is two stage implantation?

Ans. Consists of removal of prosthesis along with resection of all infected material followed by reimplantation of new prosthesis at second surgical procedure may be after at least 6 weeks.

Q.36 What are mechanisms of failure of THR?

Ans.
- Aseptic loosening—due to poor selection of patient may be mismatch of implant and bone.
- Infection—with proper antibiotics, lamilar airflow, ultraviolet rays, and proper exhaust system
- Dislocation—due to malposition of implant, impingement, sepsis, old debilated patients, etc. With posterior approach, there is higher incidence of dislocation.
- Heterotopic bone formation.
- Unstable fractures of femoral shaft.
- Breakage of component.
- Osteolysis.

Q.37 What is principle of acetabular reconstruction in revision THR?

Ans.
- Restoration of center of rotation, bony continuity and integrity.
- Contain of prosthesis and graft.
- Rigid fixation of graft.
- Proper fixation of prosthesis.

Q.38 What are options for femoral reconstruction in revision THR?

Ans. If cortex and medullary content, if age above 70 years, if there is metabolic bony disease, then cemented reconstruction should be preferred.
Otherwise cement less reconstruction should be done.

Q.39 What are results of revision THR?

Ans. With acetabular revision, cement less, ingrown sockets are useful in all types of deficiencies. With 2–7 years follow-up shows re-revision in 2.5–8% patients, migration of porous cups is seen in 17% cases, bipolar hips give high rate of migration and failures at early stage of acetabular components.

Cemented revision of socket acetabular component shows re-revision from 0–30% cases in 2–10 years follow-up.

Cemented femoral components have high rate of radiolucent rates and loosening with most cement less revisions. It depends upon stability of prosthesis, bone stock deficiency, prevention of intraoperative fractures, and type of implant chosen for specific reason and re-revision rate is still 3–10%, rigid fixation and maximal host-graft contact has given good unions.

With proper preoperative planning, with proper implant selection, use of long stems, wide exposure, preservation of proximal bone, avoidance of fracture and perforation, give better results.

Q.40 What are other options are available in failed THR?
Ans. They are:
- Hip osteotomy (femoral)—flexion, valgus, extension, varus, rotation (Sugioka) or combination of both.
- Hip arthrodesis,
- Excision arthroplasty or Girdlestone operation.

Q.41 What are the goals of hip osteotomy?
Ans. The main goal is to restore anatomy to as normal as possible and to eliminate excessive load to joint caused by abnormal joint mechanics and to change of weight-bearing axis and to relieve venous engorgement.

Q.42 What are the common conditions which treated by hip osteotomy?
Ans. Osteoarthritis, osteonecrosis, slipped capital femoral epiphysis, Legg-Calve-Perthes disease, and congenital hip dysplasia.

Q.43 When one should do hip osteotomy?
Ans. In young patients, where THR cannot be done, heavy labourers, mild symptoms, good range of movements of joint, non-obese patients.

Q.44 What are major types of osteotomies of femur?
Ans. Flexion, extension, valgus, varus, and rotational, combinations of all above.

Q.45 What is effect on limb length after hip osteotomy?
Ans. There is shortening after varus osteotomy at least 1 cm and increase in length after valgus osteotomy, if open wedge is done otherwise shortening after closed wedge valgus osteotomy.

Q.46 What are indications of varus osteotomy?
Ans. In relative valgus, neck-shaft angle more than 135°, lateral joint space disease, enlarged and congruent joint space with minimal acetabular dysplasia and spheric femoral head, the results are very good with varus osteotomy.

Q.47 What are indications for valgus osteotomy?
Ans. In relative varus neck-shaft angle, medial joint space disease, medial femoral osteophyte is rotated superiorly to weight-bearing location and thus good result.

Q.48 What are indications for flexion osteotomy?
Ans. In hip extension contracture, osteonecrosis of anterior involvement where posterior is spared with full range of extension preoperatively here the apex of osteotomy is located posteriorly so that shaft of femur is flexed and proximal femur extended.

Q.49 What are indications of extension osteotomy?
Ans. For hip flexion contracture and deficient anterior acetabular coverage, where the apex of osteotomy is located anteriorly so that the shaft of femur is extended and proximal femur is flexed.

Recurrent Dislocation of Patella

Q.1 What is habitual dislocation of patella? How it differs from recurrent dislocation of patella?

Ans. In habitual dislocation patella dislocates with each flexion of knee joint and relocated in extension. This is common in adolescent females.

In recurrent dislocation of patella-patella dislocates but not with each flexion of knee and never gets relocated in extension and associated with pain (some times).

Q.2 What are predisposing factors of recurrent dislocation of patella?

Ans. Bony-Genu valgus, patella alta, shallow groove, external tibial torsion, anteversion of femur, medial part of femur is more prominent than lateral one.

Soft tissue-tight tensor fascia lata and lateral retinaculum, patellar hypermobility, generalised ligament laxity, dastus medialis oblique, lax medial capsule.

Q.3 What is Q angle?

Ans. This is angle formed by a line drawn from ASIS to midpoint of patella and another line from tibial tuberosity, called Q angle. This is normally 90°–150° more in males.

Q.4 What is apprehension test of recurrent dislocation of patella?

Ans. There is resistance by patient on attempted to subluxate patella laterally accompanied by pain.

Q.5 What is special view of X-ray in this condition?

Ans. Skyline view is advised to know medial surface of patella and lateral condyle of femur which is taken in flexed knee joint.

Q.6 Why there is false negative patellar tap in flexion?

Ans. As in flexion synovial capsule flattens over condyles and fluid is shifted to periphery.

Q.7 What is Insall-Salvati ratio?

Ans. This is ratio of patellar articular surface to length of ligamentum patellae. Normally it is one but in patella baza it is more and in patella alta it is less than one.

Q.8 What is principle in treatment of recurrent dislocation of patella?
Ans. The axis of pull of quadriceps is shifted to laterally. It is based on:
- Those operation which change the direction of pull to normal one
- Those which create checkrein medially either proximal or distal to patella
- Those where there excision of patella is done and pull is also changed.

Q.9 What is treatment of recurrent dislocation of patella?
Ans. In children one has to take care not to injure epiphysis—so
- Campbell's operation-proximal alignment
- Hauser's operation-distal alignment [soft tissue only in children]
- Roux Gold wait operation-combined
- Excision and release of lateral tight tensor fascia lata extensively
- Corrective osteotomy for genu valgum
- Plication of capsule on medial, side
- Checkrein ligament to pull tendon on medial side.

Q.10 What is treatment of recurrent dislocation of patella in adults?
Ans. As there is degeneration of articular surface of patella excision of patella is to be done in neglected and untreated cases. Other wise Houser's bony block operation is done.

CHAPTER 24

Evaluation of Knee Joint

Q.1 What are most common causes of acute knee hemarthrosis?
Ans. ACL or posterior cruciate ligament tear, osteochondral fracture, capsule tear, lateral or medial meniscal tear.

Q.2 What are main principles of knee examination?
Ans. Precise, complete, physical examination of knee joint, systemic examination as soon as possible please do not forget to examine normal knee also.

Q.3 What are points of examination in knee case?
Ans.
- Proper and precise history of trauma, such as where was the blow whether lateral side or medial side, whether knee was extended, whether locking of joint took place, etc. History of swelling, pain description, etc.
- Inspection—attitude of limb, deformity of knee—valgus or varus, position of patella, swelling—location, local temperature, any sinuses or not.
- Gait—type of gait.
- Special tests to test effect of injury.

Q.4 What details of swelling should be noted?
Ans. Whether intra-articular or extra-articular, location of extra-articular swelling, degree of swelling—mild, moderate, severe, onset of swelling-gradual or sudden, extent and mobility of swelling.

Q.5 How general evaluation of lower extremity is done?
Ans. Ciucumferential measurement of thigh, at vastus medialis area, midpatellar area, and mid-calf
- Active and passive range of movements of knee
- Tightness of hamstrings, quadriceps, tendo-Achilles
- Hip and ankle on both sides
- Pain, type of pain and how it increases
- Neurovascular status of lower extremity.

Q.6 What radiological finding may indicate medial collateral ligament injury?
Ans. Line of calcification on medial side known as pellegrini steida lesion.

Q.7 What is significance of Segued sign? [Fracture]
Ans. This is avulsion of capsule on lateral tibia indicating ACL injury.

Q.8 How do you evaluate extensor mechanism of knee?
Ans.
- Inspection of quadriceps femoris for atrophy, tenderness and tone.
- Palpation of quadriceps and patellar tendons for continuity and tenderness
- Position (middle, subluxated or dislocated]and height of patella-patella alta-[high riding,) patella baja (low riding) with chondromalacia
- Mobility of patella with or without apprehension test
- Grating of patella with or without pain
- Tenderness at medial or lateral joint line, patellar tendon, tibial tubercle, anterior pad of fat and sizes are to be noted.

Q.9 How do you perform apprehension test? What is its significance?
Ans. Firm direct lateral force is applied to the medial border of patella to subluxate patella with some flexion of knee and if patient experiences pain and due to that he apprehends the procedure. Then this apprehension is positive test and it indicates acute or subaute subluxation of patella.

Q.10 What is abduction or valgus stress test at 30° and at 0°? What is its significance?
Ans. This test is done with 30° with supine position of patient, with one hand on lateral aspect of knee and other supporting ankle. Abduction or valgus stress is applied gently to knee and hand of ankle rotates knee externally slightly and then knee is brought to extension with repetition of gentle rocking or swinging motion. Stability of knee is tested at 30° and 0° of valgus stress. Instability at 30° flexion indicates injury to medial collateral ligament and instability at 0° indicates injury to posterior structures [capsule and posterior cruciate ligament] and medial structures.

Q.11 How adduction or varus stress test is done and what it signifies?
Ans. Patient is in supine position, knee flexed to 30°, adduction or varus stress is applied keeping one hand on medial aspect of knee and instability is tested in 30° of flexion and 0° (extension) and concluded that
- Varus instability in 30° flexion indicates that injury to lateral compartment ligaments
- Instability in extension indicates disruption of lateral capsular ligament, anterior cruciate ligament, lateral collateral ligament, iliotibial band, often posterior cruciate ligament.

Peroneal nerve is at risk in any lateral or varus injury so this should be assessed in all varus injuries without fail.

Q.12 What is Lachman test? What is its significance?
Ans. Patient is in supine position with 30° flexion, lower end of femur is stabilized by one hand and with another hand tibial upper end is given anterior force from

behind and anterior translation of tibia with soft or no endpoint is positive test, indicated injury to anterior cruciate ligament.

Q13 What is pivot shift examination?

Ans. This test is for ACL, performed under anaesthesia before surgery, with holding leg in extension, brought into flexion and when anteriorly subluxated tibia shifts or reduces to anatomical position indicates positive test.

Q.14 Why anterior drawer test is not much reliable?

Ans. When posterior horn of medial meniscus is torn or displaced, it may block anterior translation of tibia and may not give proper idea about ACL.

Q.15 What are ways of testing posterior cruciate ligament injury?

Ans.
- *Posterior drawer test:* Posterior force is applied on proximal tibia in neutral position, internal rotation and external rotation and abnormal movement of tibia indicates positive test.
- *Quadriceps active test:* Patient is in supine position, limb is relaxed with 90° flexion of knee, patient is asked to contract gently quadriceps without extension of knee, if tibia sags posteriorly and patellar ligament is directed anteriorly indicates injury to posterior cruciate ligament.

Q.16 What is Jerk test of Hughston and Losee?

Ans. This test is for assessment of anterolateral instability (ALRI) of knee joint. Patient is supine, knee is flexed to 90° flexion, lower limb is supported by examiner and internal rotation of tibia is done and valgus stress is exerted over proximal end of tibia and fibula, while knee is extended. If there is maximal subluxation of lateral femorotibial articulation at 30° of flexion and during further extension it relocates with sudden jerk then the test is positive.

Q.17 How lateral pivotal shift test of MacIntosh is done and for what?

Ans. Flex extended knee slowly, maintaining valgus and internal rotation, if there is subluxation at 30°–40° of flexion as iliotibial band passes posteriorly indicates that the test is positive. This test is for assessment ALRI instability.

Q.18 What is flexion rotation draw Noyes?

Ans. This test is also for ALRI. The leg is lifted upwards with extension of limb allowing femur to fall back and rotate externally. If there is anterolateral subluxation of tibia then the test is starting of position of test when knee is flexed, tibia moves back wards and femur rotates internally causing joint to reduce when the test is positive.

Q.19 How anterolateral drawer test is done?

Ans. Patient is supine, knee is flexed to 90° foot is rested on table anterior and internal rotation stress is applied to proximal tibia and if there is anterior and internal subluxation of lateral tibial plateau, then the test is positive.

Q.20 What is external rotation recurvation test?
Ans. This is for assessment of posterolateral instability. Patient is supine, affected limb is lifted by great toe and external rotation of tibia, posterior displacement of the tibia and recurvatum are evaluated. Peroneal nerve injury is checked.

Q.21 What is posterolateral drawer test?
Ans. Patient is supine, hip is flexed to 45°, knee is flexed 80° and the tibia is in 15° external rotation and with foot flexion posterior drawer test is performed.

Q.22 What is tibial external rotation test?
Ans. This is for posterolateral instability, external rotation of tibia on femur is tested in 30° and 90° of knee flexion in supine or prone position, taking medial border of foot as neutral position and with forceful external rotation of foot, at particular angle of flexion of knee the degree of external rotation and compared with normal limb if more than 10° external rotation is pathologic.

Q.23 How posteromedial rotary instability is diagnosed?
Ans. Posteromedial rotary instability is present when medial tibial plateau rotates posteriorly with reference to femur with medial opening of joint indicating rupture of medial collateral ligament, medial capsular ligament posterior oblique ligament, posterior cruciate ligament and major injury to the semimembranous insertions and some times anterior cruciate ligament.

Q.24 What is McMurray's test?
Ans. This is for injury to meniscus. Patient is supine, knee is acutely and forcibly flexed and with one hand posteromedial margin of joint is palpated and grasping with one hand the foot is rotated externally as far as possible keeping knee in flexion, and knee is extended slowly if painful click is felt, produced by passing of femur over tear of meniscus. This test is for medial meniscus. And same procedure is repeated but limb is rotated internally and lateral aspect of joint is palpated, if painful click is present then indicating tear in lateral meniscus.

Q.25 How the grinding test of Apley is done?
Ans. Patient is prone, knee is flexed to 90°, anterior thigh is fixed to table, foot are pulled to distract the joint and rotational strain is applied, to ligaments, painful strain indicate that the ligaments are torn. Next knee in same position, knee and foot are pressed downward and rotated as joint is slowly flexed and extended, if there is pain at joint line indicating that the meniscus is torn.

Q.26 How do you assess the site of deformity whether it is in femur or tibia in case of genu valgum?
Ans. Patient is asked to flex the knee if there is correction of valgus then it is in femur.
How? In extension flat surface of femur is in contact with tibial condyle but with full flexion more curved posterior femoral condyle comes in contact with the tibia and such deformity disappears:

- If there is partial correction of deformity occurs then the deformity is in both femur and tibia.
- If there is no correction of deformity in flexion then the deformity is mainly in tibia

PATELLOFEMORAL JOINT DISORDERS

Q.1 What are patellofemoral joint disorders?
Ans.
A. General—extensor mechanism misalignment
   Patellofemoral pain syndrome
   Runner's knee
   Chondromalacia
   Patellar subluxation or dislocation
B. Clinical varieties—patellar tendonitis [Jumper's knee]
   Quadriceps tendonitis
   Osgood Schlatter disease
   Plica
   Fat pad impingement
   Bipartite patella.

Q.2 What are typical patellofemoral complaints?
Ans.
- Anterior knee pain—most frequent complaint—pain is more after prolonged sitting in 90° flexion, repetitive stair climbing, after physical activities
- Swelling—is not routine but may be present with minimal effusion
- Catching or slipping sensations—catching may occur when underlying inflamed tissue is caught on bony prominences, or may be due to roughness of patellar surface or inflamed synovial plica.

Q.3 What are physical and radiological findings of patellofemoral problems?
Ans. The predisposing factors for patellofemoral problems are ascending, descending the stair cases, squatting and sitting for long period and some patients get pain after running jumping cutting and twisting activities.

Physical findings—pain on compression of patella, crepitations of patellofemoral joint during knee movements and apprehension on lateral displacement of patella.

X-ray picture—lateral view give idea about height of patella, and with infrapatellar view one can get better assessment about patellofemoral joint disorder. And static view may not reveal any thing as the affection is dynamic.

Q.4 What are methods of treatment of patellofemoral problems?
Ans. Initial treatment—physical therapy, such as exercises, for control of patella rather than strength and exercises for flexors of knee such as hamstrings iliotibial band, and posterior calf muscles are important rather than extensors,

strengthening hip rotators, and proprioceptive exercises are new concepts for this problem. Modification of activities.

External support—such as patellofemoral bracing or McConnel patellofemoral taping, orthotics to correct foot abnormalities, analgesic drugs (non-steroidal).

Q.5 What are surgical techniques available for this problem?

Ans. When all conservative methods fail, then following surgical procedures may be useful:
- Arthroscopic lateral release—may be useful cases where there is more pain and lateral patellar tilt.
- More extensive open procedure of lateral release with reattachment or reconstruction of medial patellofemoral ligament and vastus.
- Medialis oblique muscle along with transfer of petallar tendon attachment medially, useful for unstable patella
- Anterior advancement of tibial tuberosity—to decompress the patellofemoral joint
- Derotational osteotomy of the limb if there is rotational component
- Patelloectomy
- Excision of areas of chondromalacia
- Removal of osteochondral fractures
- Synovectomy of synovial plica
- Removal of painful accessory ossification centers.

Q.6 What makes to intervene surgically in acute dislocation of patella?

Ans. In acute dislocation of patella—there may be osteochondral fracture of patella, or lateral femoral condyle, with large fragments have to be reattached and small fragments may be removed to avoid locking in future.

In acute dislocations if there is rupture of vastus medialis obliques and medial patellofemoral ligament at their insertions then surgical repair has to be done immediately.

Q.7 What are complications after surgical procedures done for patellofemoral disorders?

Ans.
- With excessive advancement of medial structures may cause medial subluxation or dislocation
- By excessive transfer of patellar tendon may cause low lying patella with abutment with proximal tibia and may create more pain.

CHAPTER 25

Total Knee Arthroplasty

Q.1 What are major indications for total knee arthroplasty (TKR)?
Ans. Total knee arthroplasty TKR is indicated for end stage degenerative disease of knee, resulted from primary or secondary osteoarthritis of knee, avascular necrosis, and inflammatory arthropathies such as rheumatoid arthritis.

Q.2 What are nonoperative methods of treatment for osteoarthritis (OA) of knee?
Ans.
- Rest
- Orthosis, elastic knee supports or valgus unloading braces
- Nonsteroidal anti-inflammatory drugs
- Corticosteroids intra-articular injections
- Viscosupplementation
- Ambulatory aids such as cane or walker.

Q.3 What is viscosupplementation?
Ans. This is method where there is use of injectable viscoelastic preparation containing hyaluron or hylan (crosslinked hyaluronan), which is supposed to provide extra-joint protection at least for 6 months to 2 years. This drug gets absorbed within 4 weeks after injecting into knee joint. This is available in different molecular weights and injections are repeated after 6 months as there is relief of 6 months at least.

Q.4 What is function of valgus or varus unloading brace?
Ans. This brace induces valgus thrust thus decompressing medial compartment in cases of moderate degenerative disease of knee in young patients with high activity life style. The results are encouraging.

Q.5 What are surgical procedures available for OA of knee?
Ans.
- Arthroscopic debridement—done where symptoms are <1 year, with nontraumatic origin, without any deformity and mechanical symptoms.
- Osteotomy—high tibial osteotomy for varus deformity <15° with good range of movements, younger age, overweight patients, with isolated medial compartment syndrome shown on X-ray, by clinical examination.

- Distal femoral osteotomy-isolated lateral compartment involvement, and valgus deformity <15° with same indications as above
- Unicompartmental knee arthroplasty—medial or lateral
- Patellofemoral arthroplasty-arthroscopic debridement with or without release of lateral retinaculum after failure of all other methods
- Total knee arthroplasty.

Q.6 When do you advise unicompartmental arthroplasty?
Ans.
- Patient below age of 60 years
- Patient with relatively sedentary life
- Presence of knee movements more than 90°
- Flexion deformity less than 10°
- Cases of primary OA of knee
- Patients having <15° angular deformity.

The patients with above criteria can get good results with unicompartmental arthroplasty of knee.

Q.7 What are proper indications of TKR?
Ans. TKR is indicated for relief of pain, restoration of function of affected knee, achievement of good stability, and good durable reconstruction.

Q.8 What is role of surfacing of patella?
Ans.
- For inflammatory arthritis—patella should be always surfaced
- Osteoarthritis—patella surfacing has given doubtful results and there may be discomfort after resurfacing of patella in OA cases especially climbing up or down and rising from chair.

Q.9 What are approaches for TKR?
Ans.
- Straight midline incision followed by medial parapatellar capsular arthrotomy, the incisions of skin and capsule are not same so healing and sealing is better and reduces postoperative drainage and chances of infection
- Standard medial parapatellar incision with several capsular arthrotomies are used such as subvastus, splitting of vastus medialis, trivector and lateral parapatellar approach.

Q.10 What are advantages of different approaches?
Ans.
- Subvastus or southern approach—where vastus medialis obliques is elevated with medial capsulotomy, spares quadriceps tendon, quicker return of quadriceps function, and recommended in this patients.
- Vastus medialis splitting approach—here division of vastus medialis is done along its fibers at proximal two-thirds and distal one-third junction, which ends at superior medial pole of patella and incision in capsule is carried along

medial border of patella, having advantage of diminution in the number of lateral reticular releases.
- Trivector approach—involving incision of body of vastus medialis obliques, beginning 5 cm proximal to superior pole of patella extending distally along medial side of patella and muscle belly is divided. As there are three vectors of pull on the patella such as rectus femoris, vastus lateralis and vastus medialis obliques so called trivector and in this approach these three vectors are maintained. And so recovery of extension apparatus is quicker.
- Lateral parapatellar approach—straight midline skin incision, with lateral parapatellar arthrotomy used especially for severe valgus deformity, with lateral subluxation of patella, needing release of lateral retinaculum attempt is made to reduce vasculature of patella by this approach.

Q.11 In case of difficulty of eversion of patella during operation of TKR what is solution?
Ans.
- Extension of incision proximally into quadriceps tendon
- Release of adhesions in the lateral retinaculum and patellofemoreal ligament
- Peripheral osteophytes are removed
- Release of lateral retinaculum
- Tethering of medial portion of insertion of patellar ligament.

Q.12 What is mechanical axis of knee?
Ans. This is defined as line which intersects the centre of femoral head, centre of knee and ankle with purpose to reconstruct the mechanical axis with appropriate resection of tibia and femur, balancing ligamentous structures.

Q.13 What is normal alignment of distal femoral condyles in relation to femoral axis and of the tibial plateau in relation to the tibial axis?
Ans. The normal alignment of distal femoral condyles in relation to the femoral axis is approximately 9° of valgus whereas the normal alignment of tibial plateau in relation to tibial axis is approximately 3° of varus. So the final valgus is 6° facilitates creation of mechanical axis.

Q.14 What is cut of proximal tibia in relation to tibial axis?
Ans. There are two views about this:
1. Insall et al. and his followers believe that tibial resection should be created at 90° to the tibial axis in coronal plane. As varus malalignment leads to early failures and so to realign mechanical axis distal femur should be resected at 6° of valgus.
2. Hungerford et al. and others believe to resect proximal tibia in 3° of varus and distal femur in 9° of valgus, believing that this resection put the joint line parallel to the ground in coronal plane during gait.

So to conclude, it is safer to resect for 90° to accept a 2–3° variation in relation to varus or valgus to have good results.

Q.15 How do you cut proximal tibia in sagittal plane?

Ans. The proximal tibia has posterior slope of 7–10° sagittal plane so t-resection of tibia is done as follows keeping few points in mind-I-resection perpendicular to the axis where implant should have:
- Posterior slope built into articulation
- Resection of the proximal tibia with 5–7° posterior slope reconstruction of posterior slope is important in cruciate retaining of TKR.

Q.16 What are palpable landmarks to assist placement of extramedullary tibial jig?

Ans. They are tibial tubercle, tibial spine, and lateral malleolus and jig should be placed over tibial tubercle and aligned parallel with tibial spine while intersecting the medial and middle thirds of intermalleolar distance and thus lined between first and second ray of foot.

Q.17 Is it recommended to use intramedullary or extramedullary jigs for performing the distal femoral and proximal tibial resections?

Ans. Intramedullary alignment jigs offer more reliable, accurate and reproducible distal femoral resection which is quite convincing.

The proper palpatory bony landmarks allows accurate placement of extramedullary alignment jig and thus resections of tibia are made. But some times due to bowing of tibia it is not easy to put intramedullary guide properly and thus may result into slight varus or valgus malalignment.

Q.18 How the rotation of femur is determined?

Ans. The rotation of femoral component is determined by four distinct anatomic features of distal femur:
- Transepicondylar axis—which intersects the medial and lateral epicondyle representing true axis of rotation of distal femur
- The anterior or posterior axis of femur is a line from centre of trochlear groove to centre of the intercondylar notch. This axis is 90° to the transepicondylar axis
- The posterior femoral condyles are 3° rotated internally to transepicondylar axis. So with help of guide with references to posterior condyles with 3° externally rotated femoral component which is placed in line with neutral transepicondylar axis
- Tibial shaft axis is recognized as being 90° to transepicondylar axis

So while fixing TKR implant all these points are to be considered for better results.

Q.19 What methods are used for facilitating patellofemoral tracking?

Ans.
- Appropriate resection and resurfacing of patella to restore preoperative thickness.
- Placing patellar component slightly medially
- Femoral component is placed in neutral or slight external rotation

- Femoral component is place with slight lateral deviation
- Proper rotation of tibial component
- Release of patellofemoral ligament and any adhesions within lateral retinaculum
- G-release of lateral retinaculum with preservation of geniculate vessels
- Advancement and reefing of the vastus medialis obliques.

Q.20 How varus malalignment is corrected?
Ans.
- Correction of contracture by removal of peripheral osteophytes from the distal femur and proximal tibia
- Release of deep medial collateral and capsular attachment to the proximal tibia
- If no proper correction then release of superficial medial collateral ligament followed by release of pes anserinus.

These releases are taken off from the proximal tibia in addition to appropriate bony resections to align the joint properly.

Q.21 How the rotation of femoral component is determined?
Ans. Rotation of femur is best determined by locating the transepicondylar axis, which intersects the medial and lateral epicondyle.

The axis of posterior condyles is internally rotated with respect to the transepicondylar axis and so should not be used as guide to assess rotation.

Q.22 How valgus deformity is corrected?
Ans. In addition to proper bony resection in valgus knee lateral contracted tissues should be released:
- Removal of peripheral ostephytes.
- Contracture of iliotibial band is released by either release from Gerdy's tubercle versus or fractional lengthening by stab wounds or transection of IT ban at joint level.
- Posterior lateral capsule or arcuate complex is transacted with knee in full extension, protecting neurovascular structures or can be released from distal femur with flexed knee with curved osteotome.
- If still not corrected or if there is unbalancing, then gradual release of popliteus tendon and lateral collateral ligament becomes necessary of proper degrees and use of nonconstrained posterior cruciate retaining or posterior stabilized device is advisable. Posterior stabilized constrained device may be used to get stability, in cases where full release is needed.
- Rarely release of biceps may become necessary.
- Reticular release is necessary to facilitate tracking of patellofemoral articulation in valgus knee.

Q.23 How the flexion contracture of knee is corrected in TKR?
Ans. With flexion contracture—posterior stabilizing device should be used as posterior cruciate ligament is deforming force and has to be released for correction

of flexion contracture. Posterior cruciate retaining device can used with special attention to the tension within PCL. It is also suggested to do controlled release of ligament in place of total excision of PCL and to use posterior stabilized device.

It is very necessary to remove all the posterior condylar osteophytes to help in reconstruction of posterior process for any type of implant. If PCL is excised for flexion contracture posterior stabilized device can be used which substitutes PCL.

If posterior cruciate retaining device is used then the ligament has to be tethered from its insertion from proximal tibia or distal femur.

If flexion contracture is severe, then capsule has to be released from posterior femur with release of both heads of gastrocnemius has to done to get extension. If more resection of distal femur is done to increase extension space for correction of flexion contracture but there is elevation of joint line. But, if posterior cruciate retaining device is used which retains joint line which is important for function of PCL.

Q.24 What are complications of TKR?

Ans. They are getting monimal with improvement in technique and proper precautions infection, breakage of implant, dislocation of implant are few to name.

Q.25 What is new development in TKR?

Ans. Getting more and more flexion of knee. So one can sit even cross legged on the ground.

CHAPTER 26

Problems of Spine

Q.1 What are the movements of spine?
Ans.
- Flexion-normal—90°
- Extension-normal—15°. Middle finger tip reaching to PSIS
- Lateral flexion—middle finger reaching knee level
- Rotation in sitting position—normal 45° angle between shoulder and pelvis.

Q.2 What is SLR?
Ans. Described by Frost in 1881 and credited to Lessague.

Patient is supine, head is flat or on pillow, pelvis is stabilized by one hand and with the leg is elevated holding at heel, the patient is asked for any leg pain during this procedure, or any radicular pain. If this pain is there then the test is positive indicating nerve compression back pain alone is not positive test.

Q.3 What is Bowstring's sign?
Ans. Full SLR is done, knee is flexed and pressure is applied over popliteal fossa- causes radiating pain and paraesthesia on leg.

Q.4 What is reverse Leségue's test?
Ans. Patient is prone or in lateral position with unaffected side down, hip is extended and knee is flexed (opposite to SLR) in turn if there is pain due to stretching or irritation of femoral nerve indicating lumber disc prolapse and L4 nerve root is involved.

Q.5 What is Kerning's test?
Ans. Passive extension of knee is done after flexion of hip and knee, there is severe pain in involved area suggesting positive test.

Q.6 What is Milgram's test?
Ans. Patient's SLR is done up to 2 inches above ground at 30° and asked to hold for 30 seconds. If it is less than 30° then suggests disc prolapse and trapping of cord.

Q.7 What is Naffziger's test?
Ans. If there is pain, after jugular vein compression in sitting position, and if there is pain in lumber region suggests disc prolapse.

Q.8 What is sitting root test?
Ans. Patient is sitting, cervical spine is flexed, knee is extended and hip is flexed to 90°, the patient may complain of pain or may attempt to extend hip indicating nerve root compression.

Q.9 What is contralateral SLR?
Ans. The test is performed in same manner of SLR but with unaffected limb. If there is pain in affected limb then the test is positive, suggesting herniated disc with localizing extrusion usually herniation medial to nerve root.

Q.10 What are tests for sacroiliac joint affection?
Ans. They are pelvic rock test, Gaenslen's test, pump handle test, FABER's test, and forward bending and rotation test.

Q.11 What are nerve roots responsible for hip flexion?
Ans. They are—T12, L1, L2, L3

Q.12 What are nerve root values for knee extension flexion?
Ans. They are—L3, L4 for knee extension, L5-S1 for knee flexion.

Q.13 What is central cord injury?
Ans. This is incomplete spinal cord injury occurs in elderly resulting from extension injury, involving upper extremities more than lower extremities, leading to quadriplegia. 75% patients recover and become ambulatory.

Q.14 What is anterior cord syndrome?
Ans. This is defined as complete motor deficit with preservation of deep pressure and proprioception from incomplete cord injury. 50% recover with weak motor skills but only 10% become ambulatory.

Q.15 What is Brown Séquard syndrome?
Ans. Resulting from incomplete cord injury where there is ipsilateral motor loss, contralateral pain and temperature loss. Usually 90% recover.

Q.16 What is spinal shock?
Ans. It is a physiological dysfunction of nervous tissue of spinal cord after spinal cord injury after returning reflex arcs including bulbocavernosus reflex it is concluded that spinal shock is resolved.

Q.17 What is common pain pattern of herniated cervical disc?
Ans. Most common pattern of pain of cervical herniated disc is radiation into scapular area and down lateral aspect of arm up to forearm and hand.

Q.18 What are common methods of conservative treatment of cervical herniated disc?
Ans. Cervical collar, physical therapy with cervical traction, epidural steroid blocks, non-steroidal inflammatory drugs, etc. usually 50–60% is success rate, but should be tried for at least 3 months before embarking to any surgical treatment.

Q.19 What are risk factors of developing back pain?

Ans. Jobs which need heavy and repetitive lifting weight, car drivers, smokers, and obese persons are at risk of low back pain.

Q.20 How do you correlate vertebral level to neurological level?

Ans. Actually spinal cord end at lower border of L1 vertebra and accordingly the levels are changed:
- In cervical region—C1-C7- add 1
- In thoracic region—T1-T6- add 2
- In lower thoracic region—T7-T9- add 3
- T10-correspond to L1-L2, T11-correspond to L3-L4
- T12-L1 correspond to L5-S1.

Q.21 How many are intervertebral discs?

Ans. There are 23 intervertebral discs.

Q.22 How many nerve roots are there?

Ans. There are 31 nerve roots.

Q.23 What is cauda equine syndrome?

Ans. This is syndrome where there is midline herniation of disc which may compress many nerve roots (incidence-2%). The most common disc to get herniated is L4–L5. The usual symptoms of disc are not there but there may be back pain, perianal pain, difficulty of urination, increased frequency, overflow incontinence, in males recent history of impotence, leg pain with or without numbness of feet with difficulty in walking. Myelography may reveal complete block indicating large disc herniation. Treatment is only surgical intervention.

Q.24 What is clinical picture of disc herniation at level of L3–L4 (unilateral)?

Ans. Unilateral disc herniation at L3–L4 compresses L4 nerve root and there is sensory deficit at posterolateral aspect of thigh, anterior knee, and medial side of leg. Variable motor weakness in quadriceps and hip adductors. There may be changes in patellofemoral reflex.

Q.25 How does herniated disc at L4–L5 presents clinically (unilateral)?

Ans. L5 nerve root is compressed giving picture sensory deficit anterolateral leg, dorsum of foot, and great toe with motor weakness of extensor hallucis longus, gluteus medius and extensor digitorum longus and brevis. Usually no changes in reflexes are seen.

Q.26 What are physical findings with L5-S1 disc herniation [unilateral]?

Ans. There is compression of S1 nerve root producing picture of sensory deficit in lateral malleolus. Lateral foot, heel, web of 4–5 toes, motor weakness of peroneus longus, brevis, gastrocnemius soleus complex, and gluteus maximus with diminished tendo-Achilles reflex.

Problems of Spine

Q.27 What is meaning when it is named as far lateral disc herniation?

Ans. When the herniation of disc occurs lateral to spinal cord, neural foramina and produce pressure on proximal nerve root of herniated disc such as far lateral disc herniation produces L4 radiculopathy against usual pressure on L5 root [expected], conservative treatment may be tried but surgical approach should be lateral to spinal canal and facet joints.

Q.28 Which types of imaging investigations should be used in evaluation of lumbar disc disease?

Ans.
- *Myelography*—it is an invasive technique (reactions may occur in the form of headache, nausea, vomiting, localized infection, etc.), has value in previously operated spine and spinal canal stenosis if done with CT scan
- *Computerized axial tomography*—better visualization, in foraminal stenosis, lateral disc herniation, lower radium dose, no reactions, can differentiate between neural compression by bone or soft tissue, very useful in lateral or foraminal disc herniation, CT scan may miss higher lesions if limited to lower levels.
- *MRI*—can demonstrate intraspinal tumors, better anatomical details of neural elements are seen, better visualization of soft tissue affection, but can visualize bony details like CT scan.
- *Bone scan*—when there is suspicion of bony disease such as neoplasms, infection, trauma, or arthritic problems which are better confirmed.

Q.29 What are surgical operations done in lumbar disc disease?

Ans.
- Usual disc removal by laminectomy by midline incision, success rate is 93% for relief of leg pain and 80% relief of low back pain.
- Microlumbar disc excision [Hijikata] done with operating microscope, laminae are not removed. This requires less dissection of tissues, less reactive scar. But results are similar to open disc operations.
- *Percutaneous automated discectomy*—cannula is placed into disc and disc material is aspirated. This is not widely used technique.
- *Endoscopic technique*—disc material is removed by an endoscope which is placed in the disc by foraminal approach, very useful for far lateral disc herniation.
- Microendoscopic discecetomy (MED)—by posterior approach very much identical to microdiscectomy by docking cannula under fluoroscope guidance, laminectomy, removal of ligament and disc is done. Migrated disc also can be removed.

Q.30 What are complications of lumbar disc surgery?

Ans. They are:
Cauda equine syndrome, thrombophlebitis, pulmonary embolism, wound infection, pyogenic spondylitis, postoperative discitis, dural tears, nerve root

injury, cerebral spinal fluid fistula, laceration of abdominal vessels and injury to abdominal viscera.

Q.31 What is spinal canal stenosis?
Ans. This is an abnormal narrowing of osteoligamentous vertebral canal or vertebral foramina causing compression over dural sac and/or nerve root. This most common cause of leg pain in elderly people unless and proved other wise. Disc herniation is rare cause of spinal canal stenosis.

Q.32 What is normal diameter of canal in the spine?
Ans.
Cervical— 15–22 mm
Thoracic— 15–22 mm
Lumbar— L1–L3–15–24 mm
L4–l5–16–28 mm.

Q.33 How do you classify lumbar canal stenosis?
Ans. Congenital-idiopathic, achondroplastic, acquired-degenerative central canal, peripheral canal, lateral recess, nerve root canal, degenerative spondylolisthesis, post-traumatic, post-chemonucleolysis, iatrogenic such as after laminectomy, after fusion, miscellaneous-Paget's disease, diffuse interstitial skeletal hypertrophy.

Q.34 Which is most common cause of canal stenosis?
Ans. Acquired degenerative spinal canal stenosis in elderly people.

Q.35 What pathology is involved with spinal canal stenosis?
Ans. Spinal canal stenosis involves three joint complex of disc facet joint and intervertebral disc which undergoes degenerative changes significantly, leading to collapse of disc and leading to facet arthritis which in turn leads to narrowing of neural foramina, which is narrowed with extension than flexion of lumbar vertebrae.

Q.36 What is clinical picture of spinal canal stenosis?
Ans. Presenting with low back pain, and stiffness which worsens with changes in weather, relieved with rest, aggravated with over activity. There is buttock discomfort, tightness or burning induced by walking pain increased with extension of spine. There may be urinary discomfort.

Q.37 What are radiological findings in case of spinal canal stenosis?
Ans. CT scan and MRI, both can give better clues for this. If sagittal diameter is 10–12 mm then it is true stenosis.

Q.38 What is treatment of spinal canal stenosis?
Ans. *Conservative*—vigorous physiotherapy, changing postural habits, stretching and strengthening tight lumbar and lower extremity muscles, TNS may be useful,

epidural steroids may help, and support by braces may minimizes lumbar lordosis and thus there may be relief.

Surgical—when conservative line fails and pain is more severe and acute, intractable pain, surgical intervention is indicated which includes removal of lamina, ligamentum flavum, spinous process, lateral recess, arthritic spurs taking care not to injure face joints.

Q.39 What are complications after decompression of spinal canal stenosis?
Ans. Instability, dural tears, infection, arachnoiditis, nerve root injury, epidural scarring.

Q.40 What are indications of fusion of spine?
Ans. Indicated for unstable fractures of spine [after disc or spinal canal stenosis operations] spondylosis and spondylolisthesis with symptoms, recurrent disc herniations, disc degeneration.

Q.41 What different ways of lumbar spine fusion?
Ans. This can be done either posteriorly or anteriorly with or without instrumentation. Bone grafts are used in both methods.

Posterior—posterolateral fusion-bone graft is placed on decorticated transverse processes, lateral facet joints, and sacral ala.

Posterior interbody (Cloward)—bone graft is placed in the intervertebral space, by posterior approach.

Spinal instrumentation enhances rate of fusion especially after spondylolisthesis when posterior pedicle screws connected with rods.

Anterior—done by trans or retroperitoneal, bone grafts are placed anteriorly for anterior inter body fusion, may be accompanied by posterior instrumentation.

Threaded titanium cages have been developed which are placed in the disc space either by anterior or posterior approaches. Endoscopic techniques are being developed to do lumbar fusion.

Q.42 What is spondylolysis?
Ans. This describes defect in pars interarticular is usually affect lumbar spine.

Q.43 What is spondylolisthesis? What are types of the same?
Ans. Means slipping forward upper vertebral segment over lower vertebra may be due to bilateral defects in pars interarticular is at level of affection [usual incidence-5% of general population.

The types are as follows:

Dysplastic—there is congenital defect in inferior defect of L5, or superior facet of S1, with elongation of pars interarticularis.

Isthmic—this is seen in sportsmen in diving, wrestling, and gymnastics where there is repetitive hyperextension causing shear of posterior elements.

Degenerative—due to degenerative disease and seen in elderly people traumatic-due to trauma.

Pathologic—due to existing pathology in the spine such as tumor.

Q.44 What is Scotty dog sign and Greyhound sign?

Ans. This is radiological sign seen on lateral X-ray in especially isthmic type, actual defect in pars interarticular is appears like collar around Scotty dog's neck.

Greyhound sign—seen in dysplastic type, on X-ray it appears as elongated pars interarticular is of L5.

Q.45 What is stress reaction?

Ans. This is phase seen before appearance of bony defect, seen on X-ray as sclerosis or elongation of pars interarticular is, seen often on contralateral side in unilateral spondylosis.

Q.46 How do you measure percentage of slip?

Ans. This is measured as distance between posterior border of body of L5 and posterior border of body S1 as percentage of anteroposterior diameter of S1. The slip angle is measured drawing a perpendicular line along posterior border of sacrum and another line parallel to inferior end plate of L5. The angle which is formed by intersection of these two lines will be slip angle.

Q.47 What are grades of spondylolisthesis?

Ans. *According to meyerding they are as follows:*
Grade 0—no anterior slip of upper vertebra on lower
Grade I—slippage 1–25%
Grade II—slippage 26–50%
Grade III—slippage 51–75%
Grade IV—complete anterior dislocation of upper over lower vertebral body.

Q.48 What are types of treatment of spondylolisthesis of Grade I?

Ans. Grade I-restriction of heavy activities, strengthening exercises of muscles, support of back by corset or so, and monitoring the symptoms. If no relief then with further investigations like CT scan confirmation of defect and bone grafting with internal fixation of spine is good solution.

Q.49 What is Gill procedure?

Ans. Removal of loose laminar fragment, fibrocartilagenous pars defect, may be followed by fusion of spine.

Q.50 What are three columns of Denis?

Ans. Posterior column—spinous process, lamina, facets, pedicles, and posterior ligamentous structures.

Middle column—posterior vertebral body, posterior annulus fibrosus, posterior longitudinal ligament

Anterior column—anterior vertebral body, anterior annulus fibrosus, anterior longitudinal ligament.

Q.51 What are different types of treatment as per grades?

Ans. *Grade II (25-50% slippage)*—proper monitoring, spot lateral X-ray, posterolateral fusion of L5-S1 with symptoms of persistent back pain, and /or neurological deficit.

Grade III (50-75%)—choice of treatment is of posterolateral fusion, L4 also included in fusion, may be combined with anterior fusion.

Grade IV—fusion of spine with or without instrumentation with or without reduction.

Q.52 What are current indications and methods of reduction?

Ans. With neurological deficit, nerve root decompression before reduction. Reduction can be achieved by halo skin traction with or without pelvic extension, segmental posterior instrumentation and posterolateral bone grafting, with or without anterior or posterior inter body fusion.

Q.53 What is conus medullar is?

Ans. It is end of spinal cord may be at level of first or second lumbar vertebra.

Q.54 What is cauda equina?

Ans. Cauda equina is below conus medullar is filled with motor and sensory nerve roots. There is more room for these roots at this level so less likely injured are not tethered to same degree as in the spinal cord.

Q.55 What are common posterior instrumentation methods for spinal stabilization?

Ans. Pedicle screws, multiple hooks and rod-third generation instrumentation to increase translation and rotational stability.
Luque—rod with sublaminar wiring.

Q.56 What are stages of disc prolapse?

Ans. Normal bulge, protrusion, extrusion and sequestration.

Q.57 What is chemonucleolysis?

Ans. Injection of chymopapain into disc causes dissolution of disc and reduces pressure in the disc.

Q.58 What is role of epidural steroids?

Ans. Reduces acute pain, inflammation, reduces fibrosis, wear and tear, usually used in acute low back pain.

Q.59 What are causes of failed back syndrome?

Ans. Incomplete removal of disc or failure to remove, stenosis, scarring, foreign body, nerve injury, adhesive arachnoiditis, overlooking of second lesion or further extrusion.

Q.60 What are causes of isthmic spondylolisthesis?

Ans.
- Birth fracture of pars
- Stress fracture
- Failure of fusion of laminae
- Hereditary
- Impingement of articular process—pinch like compression of L5 between L4 and sacrum.

Q.61 What is lumbar index?

Ans. This is degree of trapezoidal deformation of lumbar vertebra. Height of posterior border divided by height of anterior border and multiplied by 100 is lumbar index.

Q.62 What is Ulman's sign?

Ans. Seen on X-ray in lateral view when inferior surface of sacrum projected to anterior inferior border of L5.

Q.63 What are principles of treatment of spondylolisthesis in children?

Ans. When slip increases in few years, up to 15% of slip no treatment, but if the slip is more than 50% with or without symptoms surgery is indicated, surgery is also indicated in persistent symptoms, progressive slip, fusion is done to relieve pain and decompression is done if neurological deficit is present.

Q.64 What is role of reduction in lysthesis?

Ans. It is advisable to reduce in displacements less than 50%.

CHAPTER 27

Tuberculous Infection of Spine

Q.1 What are common sites of vertebral column which are affected by tuberculosis?
Ans. In order of frequency they are—dorsal (42%) lumbar (26%), cervical (12%) and dorsolumbar (12%), lumbosacral including sacrum.

Q.2 What are parts of vertebra which are affected by tuberculosis?
Ans.
- Paradiscal
- Central
- Appendical
- Anterior.

Q.3 What is first sign of involvement of spine?
Ans. Paradiscal—narrowing of intervertebral disc space followed by bony destruction.

Q.4 Is Pott's spine primary or secondary lesion?
Ans. Pott' spine is always secondary lesion of primary somewhere else such as lungs or lymph glands of abdomen.

Q.5 What are radiological features of Pott's spine?
Ans. Narrowing of disc space, bony destruction, shadow of paravertebral abscess in thoracic below D4. Appearance of bird nest, upper thoracic—V shaped shadow, thoracic region there is tense paravertebral abscess giving saw tooth appearance, collapse of one vertebra giving to gibbus, followed by curve leading to kyphosis with or without scoliosis.

Q.6 How does kyphosis develops in Pott's spine?
Ans. It is destruction of disc space to start then destruction of adjacent bony margins of vertebra, followed by destruction of vertebral body, collapse, wedging of body and posterior convex curve is developed leading to kyphosis.

Q.7 What are sites of tracking of Pott's abscess?
Ans. Pus of Pott's abscess can tikle down as follows.
Above diaphragm—along the intercostals vessels anywhere along chest wall.

Below diaphragm—to renal angle, Petit's triangle, inguinal fossa, Scarpa's triangle [femoral triangle] and posterior aspect of thigh.

Q.8 What are other investigations other than plain X-ray of spine?
Ans.
- CT scan—can reveal Pott's disease of posterior spinal disease, sacral lesions, craniovertebral lesions, lytic lesion of sacroiliac joint. This is better method to assess any bony lesion.
- MRI—can give better idea about disease of posterior element, vertebral appendages, this is good for assessing bony as well as soft tissue affection.
- Myelography—very useful in cases of spinal tumor syndrome where there is no clear radiological evidence of bony lesion, and in cases of multiple vertebral lesions, in cases where there is no recovery after decompression operation. This is to determine level of obstruction.

Q.9 What is classification of Pott's paraplegia?
Ans. Paraplegia due to tuberculosis is divided into two major groups-[Griffiths, Sodden and Roaf-1935]
- Group A—early onset paraplegia, which comes during active phase of disease, within first 2 years after onset, may be due to inflammatory edema, tuberculosis granulation tissue, tubercular abscess, tuberculous caseous tissue and rarely ischemia of cord.
- Group B—late onset of paraplegia, which appears many years[more than 2] after disease has persisted in the vertebral column, usually due to reactivation of disease similar to early onset of paraplegia or mechanical pressure over the cord such as due to internal gibbus, stenosis of vertebral canal, or severe deformity, tuberculous debris, seqeuestra from vertebral body or disc, etc. may be associated with apparently healed disease.

Other way of classification by staging [Goel-1967, Tuli-1985, Kumar-1988]

Stage I—patient is unaware of any motor weakness but attending physician detects plantar extensor or ankle clonus with or without brisk tendon reflexes.

Stage II—patient has clumsiness or spasticity or jumpiness of limbs while walking but manages to walk, there are signs of spastic paresis.

Stage III—non-ambulatory because of weakness of muscles, bedridden, paraplegia in extension, sensory deficit if any less than 50%.

Stage IV—flexor spasms, paraplegia in flexion, flaccid and no control over sphincters and sensory deficit more than 50%, this is terminal stage created by progressive compressive myelopathy may be associated with arachnoiditis.

Q.10 Which system recovers first?
Ans. Motor system recovers first and then sensory system recovers.

Q.11 What is spinal tumor syndrome?
Ans. A small tuberculoma or extradural granuloma causing neurological complications without any visible changes on X-ray of vertebra are labeled as spinal tumor syndromes.

Q.12 What are causes of neurological complications of Pott's spine?
Ans. They are:
- Inflammatory—edema, abscess, granuloma, caseating material.
- Mechanical—debris, sequestra, constriction
- Intrinsic—prolonged stretching of cord, dislocations,
- Spinal tumor syndrome—diffused extradural granuloma.

Q.13 What are different methods of treatment of Pott's paraplegia?
Ans. Conservative—bed rest and 4 drug therapy for 3-4 weeks and then if there is no recovery, patient is subjected to operation, where the principle is to decompress or to relieve the cord from compression by
- Costotransversectomy
- Anterolateral decompression
- Anterior decompression
- Laminectomy—when disease is restricted to posterior part of vertebra, appendages, or spinal tumor syndrome.

Q.14 What is costotransversectomy?
Ans. This is indicated where there is frank tubercular abscess, with semicircular incision 6 cm away from midline, first transverse process is removed from its base then after proper exposing the rib, it is excised up to 8 cm and abscess is sucked to get decompression. If the pus is not found, then 2nd adjacent rib is also removed with its transverse process to expose pus or abscess.

Q.15 What are indications of decompression for Pott's paraplegia?
Ans. *Absolute indications:*
- Paraplegia with onset during conservative treatment
- Paraplegia getting worse or remaining stationary in spite of treatment
- Complete loss of motor power for one month in spite of treatment
- Paraplegia with uncontrollable spasticity when it becomes difficult to keep patient in bed which may cause necrosis of skin
- Severe paraplegia of rapid onset which may be due to severe pressure
- Severe flaccid paraplegia, paraplegia in flexion, complete sensory loss, complete loss of motor power for more than 6 months.

Relative indications:
- Recurrent paraplegia
- Paraplegia in old age
- Painful paraplegia
- Paraplegia with urinary tract infection and stone.

Rare indications:
- Posterior spinal disease
- Spinal tumor syndrome
- Severe paralysis secondary to cervical spine disease
- Severe cauda equina paralysis.

Q.16 What is middle path regimen?

Ans. Rest, antitubercular drugs, regular monitoring by X-ray and ESR—every 3– 6 months, gradual mobilization and aspiration of abscesses with local installation of INH or streptomycin. If there are no signs of recovery for 4–6 weeks then decompression has to be carried out by excisional surgery of posterior spinal diseases, debridement by operation with or without spinal fusion (anterior or posterior).

Q.17 What is anterolateral decompression?

Ans. This is also known as lateral rachotomy [Capener-1933] as the spine is approached from its lateral side which affords the access to the front and side of the cord allowing to do decompression by removing bony spurs, granulation tissue, sequestra, or thorough evacuation of abscess which is done by removing 2-4 ribs with their transverse processes with some anterolateral part of body of vertebra at the level of lesion.

Q.18 What is anterior decompression?

Ans. Through transthoracic approach either by extrapleural or transpleural approach the abscess is reached and drained, debris is removed, granulation tissue is removed and decompression is achieved (Kirkaldy-1965, Hodgson-1956). Anterior spinal fusion is done by using pieces of excised rib (vertically), put in the gap created by removal of diseased vertebra usually grafts are more in length and the gap is widened by forceps grafts are put and forceps are released and thus the grafts are under optimum compression so as to get early fusion.

Q.19 What is natural course of healing of pott's spine?

Ans. If treated properly stable fibrous ankylosis, when bone grafts are used then stable bony fusion.

Q.20 What fate of cored if decompression is not done?

Ans. Loss of neurons, loss of myelin and there may be syringomyelic changes.

Q.21 What is etiology of recurrences?

Ans. Severe kyphosis, reactivation of disease in apparently healed lesion, resistant organisms.

Q.22 What are signs of healing on X-ray?

Ans. Good mineralisation of vertebrae, intervertebral space is filled with fibrous tissue or if operated by osseous tissue, regeneration of boby.

Q.23 What are good prognostic signs?

Ans. If the lesion is of shorter duration, partial involvement, type A—paraplegia, slow onset, younger age group, good general condition, active stage of disease, and less than 60° kyphosis, then there are good chances of recovery.

Q.24 What are presentations of psoas abscess?

Ans. Lump in iliac fossa, false hip flexion deformity, and tracking of abscess from anterior side to front of thigh or posteriorly up to tendo-achilles.

Q.25 What is cause of narrowing of disc space in paradiscal lesion?

Ans. Disc has no blood supply and lower margin of upper vertebra and upper margin of lower vertebra has good blood supply and thus organisms are carried to avascular region and that is why disc is first to get involved and there is narrowing of disc space.

Q.26 What is difference of lesions of spine in adults and children?

Ans. In children—bodies are affected as anterior artery supplying blood is in the centre.

In adults—there are peripheral arteries supplying lower and upper margins of vertebrae and thus disc space is involved first.

28 CHAPTER

Poliomyelitis

Q.1 What is poliomyelitis?
Ans. The poliomyelitis virus is an enterovirus, when contracted, anterior horn cells of spinal cord are destroyed with permanent loss of motor power.

Q.2 What strains of poliomyelitis are there?
Ans.
 i. Brunhide
 ii. Lensing
 iii. Leon.

Q.3 What type is polio virus?
Ans. RNA type and enterovirus.

Q.4 What types of clinical poliomyelitis are there?
Ans.
- Abortive type—brief illness with anorexia, nausea, vomiting, headache, sore throat, diarrhoea, cough, and pharyngeal exudates.
- Non-paralytic poliomyelitis—similar symptoms like abortive type with more intense headache, nausea, vomiting with soreness and stiffness of muscles esp. of back and trunk and extremities.
- Paralytic poliomyelitis—there are all symptoms like above two types with weakness or paralysis of trunk and extremities,there are two types:
   i. Spinal—which is most common involving neck, trunk and extremities
   ii. Bulbar type—involving one or two cranial nerves or there may be combination of spinal and bulbar type.

Q.5 How do you manage poliomyelitis case during convalescent to prevent deformity?
Ans. Rest to part, avoiding overexertion, support by splint (plaster or ready made) is given to prevent spasms. Lower limbs are kept in abduction, neutral rotation at hip. Knee are flexed up to functional position avoiding giving even intramuscular injections and Hubbard tank baths are used.

Q.6 How does polio virus spread?
Ans. Spread of virus from person to person via decal and oral routes.

Q.7 What kind of vaccines are available to prevent poliomyelitis? Which one is the best?

Ans. There are two types of vaccines:
1. Oral-living attenuated virus (Sabin)
2. Injectable-killed virus [Salk].

The current concept is that to start with-first dose of killed virus as this minimizes vaccine induced polio as it is seen in oral vaccine sometimes.

Q.8 How gradation of muscle power is done?

Ans. There are 5 grades of muscle power which is assessed as follows:

Grade 0—no muscle twitch at all.

Grade I—muscle twitching is felt without any useful motion.

Grade II—muscle moves joint but after elimination of gravity

Grade III—Full range of joint motion against gravity

Grade IV—motion of joint by muscle against gravity and some resistance.

Grade V—normal muscle power.

Q.9 Does muscle power loses with growing age?

Ans. Yes, with growing age the muscle loses its power at least by 5%.

Q.10 What are muscles needed to keep knee from giving way during walking?

Ans. Quadriceps is first and important muscle to keep knee stable but in absence of this muscle gluteus maximus and soleus muscles take its place.

Q.11 Does poliomyelitis affects growth? How?

Ans. Yes it does, when there is no normal muscle activity across a joint, the cartilage cells of physis are not stimulated to grow normally and short leg is the result.

Q.12 How does muscle weakness of poliomyelitis result in deformity?

Ans. Deformities from muscle weakness can be result of imbalance of muscles or of fibrosis of dead muscles. Lack of muscle pull can also change the shape of bone.

Q.13 How does muscle become fibrotic?

Ans. When nerve to muscle dies, the muscle gradually becomes atrophic and is replaced by fibrosis, which can work as tough band preventing joint from going through its full range of motion.

Q.14 What are method of treatment to correct contractures?

Ans. In young children below age of 3 years, exercises may be sufficient to over come contractures.

If child is old, contracture becomes stiffer which has to be treated by serial castings and wedging.

If child is more old and if other treatments have not responded then soft tissue release can be done to correct deformities or bony osteotomies has to done for correction.

Q.15 what are principles of tendon transfer?
Ans. Muscle to be transferred should have power of at least grade IV as during transfer it loses power by one grade.

Phasic transfers are preferred, neurovascular functions should be normal, paratenon and sheaths should not be removed, range of excursion of tendon should be normal to the muscle to be replaced.

Q.16 What is phasic and non-phasic transfer?
Ans. Phasic—when transferred in the same phase of gait
Non-phasic—when transferred in other phase of gait.

Q.17 What are muscles of lower limb which are commonly affected in polio?
Ans. These are tibialis anterior, peronei, quadriceps, glutei and lastly triceps.

Q.18 What are causes of pelvic obliquity?
Ans. Suprapelvic obliquity—due to scoliosis
At the level of pelvis—ill development of pelvis
Infrapelvic—due to tight iliotibial band, limb length discrepancy.

Q.19 What are ill-effects of pelvic obliquity?
Ans. There is flexion abduction external rotation at hip, genu valgum, flexion contracture at knee, varus of foot, external tibial torsion, lordosis, scoliosis

Q.20 How do you treat pelvic obliquity? Describe Yount's and Souttar's operations.
Ans. Sectioning of IT band by Souttar's or Yount's operation.

Yount's operation—open or closed tenotomy of iliotibial band Some times it is necessary to excise small piece of IT band to avoid recurrence.

Souttar's operation—anterior soft tissue release through an iliofemoral incision cutting or stripping all muscles from iliac crest mainly flexors and abductors.

Q.21 How quadriceps is strengthened?
Ans. When quadriceps is weak and hand to knee gait then it is necessary to do transfer of biceps femoris tendon to quadriceps make quadriceps more strong (Caldwell's operation).

Q.22 How do you treat by bony operation the genu recurvatum deformity?
Ans. A supracondylar corrective osteotomy can be done for this.

Q.23 How do you prescribe caliper in foot deformity?
Ans. Caliper with T strap on correction side and double iron bars on deformity side.

Q.24 How do you treat calcaneus foot?
Ans. This is dynamic deformity and very difficult to treat this. In skeletally immature foot aim is to correct deformity without damaging bone tendon

transfers to calcaneum to get plantar flexion are done such transfer of tibialis posterior and peroneii or if these are weak then tibialis anterior to calcaneum (Peabody).

In skeletal mature foot, plantar fasciotomy with Elimsle, reversal Lambrinudi's or triple arthrodesis is done to stabilize foot.

Q.25 How do you treat weak tibialis anterior with dropping of head of first metatarsal?
Ans. By transferring extensor hallucis longus to neck of 1st metatarsal, with fusion of interphalangeal joint of great toe (Modified Jones operation).

Q.26 What is Irwin's procedure?
Ans. Irwin's procedure consists of Steindler's fasciotomy, modified Jones operation, triple arthrodesis and transfer of peroneus longus and brevis to calcaneus for calcaneo-cavo-valgus-foot.

Q.27 What is triple arthrodesis?
Ans. When there is unstable foot after poliomyelitis and the foot is skeletally matured or there is dynamic foot deformity, then three joints—talocalcaneal, talonavicular and calcaneocuboid joints—are fused in functional position and make the foot stable.

Q.28 What are different methods of doing triple arthrodesis?
Ans. Ryerson's method, Hoke's method, Dunn's method, Lambrinudi's method (where talus is anchored to cuneiform bones after excising navicular bone to correct equines deformity), reversal Lambrinudi operation.

Q.29 What are different methods of subtalar arthrodesis ?
Ans. They are:
- Grice's operation—extra-articular arthrodesis is done in skeletally immature foot
- Dennyson-Fulford fusion
- Batchelor's arthrodesis.

Q.30 When hip gets dislocated in poliomyelitis?
Ans. That can happen in weak abductors and extensors, coax valga and femoral anteversion with pelvic obliquity.

Q.31 What is bone block procedure?
Ans. Extra-articular bone grafts are placed to control certain movements of joint esp. when tendon transfer cannot be done due to weak muscles.

Q.32 What deformities are produced at shoulder in polio?
Ans. Deltoid paralysis, serratus anterior paralysis, (abductor insufficiency).

Q.33 What is type of muscle involvement in poliomyelitis?
Ans. It is patchy, irregular, asymmetric.

29 CHAPTER

Volkmann's Ischemic Contracture

Q.1 What is Volkmann's ischaemic contracture (VIC)?
Ans. Described by Richard von Volkmann in 1881, about the contracture and paralysis caused by tissue damage following compartment syndromes. There is ischaemic muscle damage and characteristic position of hand after forearm compartment syndromes, commonly after tide bandaging of the upper extremity.

Q.2 What are five Ps of compartment syndrome?
Ans. Pain, pallor paralysis, paraesthesia and pulselessness.

Q.3 What are five most common causes of compartment syndromes?
Ans. Fracture, soft tissue injury, arterial injury, prolonged compression of limb and burns.

Q.4 How the pressure is measured in compartment in syndromes?
Ans. Many methods are available:
- White side—infusion technique
- Matsen—similar infusion technique but continuous monitoring by infusion pump and blood pressure transducer
- Mubarak's wick catheter technique—which measures directly depression
- Striker method—simple and reliable device.

Q.5 Which nerve is most commonly involved? Why?
Ans. The median nerve is commonly involved as it runs in the centre of (its branch) ellipsoid Seddon's area and so there is profound ischaemia.

Q.6 What is differential diagnosis of Volkmann's contracture?
Ans.
- Degeneration of muscle following sepsis
- Haemophilia with bleeding in forearm
- Drug induced compartment syndromes such as alcohol.

Q.7 How many entities are after Volkmann?
Ans. Volkmann's canal in bone, Volkmann's test, Volkmann's contracture.

Q.8 Describe the deformity of VIC.

Ans. Flexion of wrist, extension of fingers at metacarpophalangeal joints (MCP) flexion at interphalangeal joint (IP), pronation of forearm and may be flexion of elbow.

Q.9 How do you describe Seddon's area of affection?

Ans. There is infarct of muscles in the form of an ellipsoid where the axis is in the line of anterior interosseous artery and the central line is a middle of forearm, called Seddon's area. The most damaged muscles are flexor digitorum profundus (FDP) and flexor pollicis longus (FPL) and the greatest damage is at the centre.

Q.10 What is a muscle sequestrum?

Ans. There is muscle degeneration in the centre with cellular activity followed by fibrosis at periphery with sheath of fibrous tissue. This degeneration of muscle is the sequestrum.

Q.11 When one should start active treatment?

Ans. After degeneration of muscle, there is good recovery of extension muscles with few flexors and the nerve within 3 to 6 months so one should wait at least for 3 months before starting any active treatment or surgery.

Q.12 What is Seddon's operation?

Ans. In acute and subacute phase, Sedddon has recommended excision of necrosed and damaged muscle and tissue, to make a space for regeneration of tissue thereof. If this operation is done at early stage, chances of recovery is very well.

Q.13 How do you treat case of VIC?

Ans. Conservative treatment—physiotherapy—active and passive to make the joints supple.

Operative treatment:
- Garre's operation—shortening of the bone by 2–2.5 cm.
- Maxpage's operation—there is sliding of muscles from common flexor origin from medial epicondyle, muscles are erase from the bone.
- Tendon transfers—active available tendons are transferred
- Muscle transplanting
- Grafting of nerves
- Reconstructive procedures.

Q.14 What is most recent trend of treatment of VIC?

Ans. By application of JESS distractor – by application of external fixator, slow and gradual distraction of fibrosed muscles and tendons, give good result. JESS distractor means Dr Joshi's Controlled External Stabilising System.

CHAPTER 30

Non-union

Q.1 What is non-union?
Ans. After stipulated time, union of the bone stops, not showing any signs of union is labeled non-union. In adults this is approx 3 months.

Q.2 What is a difference between delayed union and non-union?
Ans. *Delayed union*—there are some signs of healing of bone are there but it is delayed more than stipulated time. This may lead to union.
Non-union—this is a definite stage of stoppage of union of bone with some definite signs.

Q.3 What are different types of non-union?
Ans. *Hypertrophic*—Hypertrophy of bony ends medullary canal may be open at both ends but usually obliterated, there is sclerosis weight seen at fracture-ends with sclerosed callus gap in between two fragments is seen-elephant's foot appearance, requires fixation and horse hoof. Clinically—there are few abnormal movements at fracture side.
Hypervascular or hypertrophic (horse hoof)
- Hypertrophic non-unions are rich in callus and have a rich blood supply in the ends of the fragments.
- They result from insecure fixation or premature weight bearing in a reduced fracture whose fragments are viable.

Oligotrophic non-unions: These are not hypertrophic, and callus is absent; they typically occur after major displacement of fracture, distraction of fragments, or internal fixation w/o accurate apposition of fragments.

Avascular or atrophic: Ends of the fragments have become osteoporotic and atrophic; the non-union is inert and incapable of biologic reaction; there is poor blood supply to the ends of the fragments; these are typically seen in tibial fracture treated by plate and screws; these are usually final result when intermediate fragments are missing and scar tissue that lacks osteogenic potential is left in their place.

Q.4 What are the causes of different types of non-union?
Ans.
- Hypertrophy—improper and insufficient immobilization
- Oligotrophic—no rigid retention
- Atrophic—hypovascularity of bony ends

Q.5 What are the causes of atrophic non-union?
Ans.
- Infection—may be after operation
- Severe comminution
- Open contaminated fractures and improper and delayed treatment.

Q.6 What are the treatment modes available for infected non-union?
Ans. Rheinländer's method—debridement, bone graft, skin cover and exterior fixation

Harmon's posterolateral bone grafting—useful when there is no anterior skin cover of especially tibia.

Friedlander's techniques—debridement, stabilisation and open bone grafting.

Ilizarov's ring fixation—gradual and slow distraction gives good regeneration of bone.

Q.7 What is a bone graft?
Ans. It is a bone transplant used for stability and repair of bone in cases of where bone gap is present with the purpose osteogenesis.

Q.8 What are clinical applications of bone grafts?
Ans. For spinal fusion, arthrodesis, enhancement of fracture healing and repair of pseudoarthrosis, reconstructive surgery, oral and maxillary surgery.

Q.9 From where bone grafts are taken commonly?
Ans. Cortical—fibula—upper 2/3

Cancellous—iliac crest, olecranon, upper end of tibia, head of femur (after excision). Medial surface of tibia, posterior should be iliac spine, upper end of tibia, femoral condyle.

Corticocancellous—metaphysis of tibia, iliac crest.

Q.10 How does the cortical and cancellous bone grafts get incorporated?
Ans. Cortical bone graft—never incorporated, absorption of the graft and slow replacement by new bone by surrounding tissue and bone. It takes long time as much as two years.

Cancellous bone graft—it may get incorporated by providing morphogenic protein, lattices network for neo-osteosynthesis and creeping substitution.

Q.11 What is Phemister bone grafting?
Ans. This was described by Phemister and modified by Forbe.

Fracture side is not opened and disturbed, but corticocancellous bone grafts are laid proximal and distal to the fracture which has gone into delayed union by fibrous union.

Q.12 What is a law of distraction compression osteosynthesis?

Ans. According to Ilizarov (1951), "When steady traction in the line of tension put on the living tissue then there is a new tissue or bone formation".

Q.13 What is role of compression on bone grafting?

Ans. According to Wolff—optimum compression between bony ends may induce neo- osteogenesis leading to bony healing.

Q.14 What are the latest methods for treatment of non-union?

Ans.
- Phoe's technique—vascularised bone grafts
- Electrostimulation—magnetic
- Percutaneous bone marrow grafting
- Pulverised bone grafts with percutaneous bone marrow grafts.

Q.15 What is piezoelectric effect in union?

Ans. Each bone acts as a dipole and on break in continuity of bone there occurs positive and negative charge around the surface of bone and this causes increased osteogenic activity.

Q.16 What is fate of bone graft?

Ans. Though it is not established but usually it follows serially—necrosis, mitosis, revascularisation, osteogenesis, remodeling and growth.

Q.17 Does bone grow back at donor site?

Ans. No, bones do not grow back at donor site.

Q.18 What is osteoid?

Ans. Osteoid is non-mineralised precursor of bone which is formed by osteoplasties induced from precursor cells by fracture hematoma. Osteoid consist of type I collagen, numerous miscellaneous materials including glycoproteins and other proteins and when osteoid gets matured calcium hydroxyapatite crystals are deposited, giving new strength to new bone.

Q.19 What are processes by which bone grafting lead to bone formation?

Ans. Osteogenesis is found only in autografts where the cellular elements remain viable. Osteogenesis is new bone formation from viable stem or osteoprogenitor cells which retain capacity to differentiate into bone forming cells. This is seen in vascularised bone graft of fibula which gives better results.

Osteoinduction is the ability of the graft to induce stem cells to differentiate into mature osteoblasts and osteocytes, this should be present for osteogenesis and seen in autografts.

Osteoconduction is the ability of the graft to serve as framework on which the host cells can form living bone. Allograft is classic example of osteoconductivity.

Q.20 What are three stages of bone healing?
Ans.
1. Inflammatory stage—which is for first 1-3 days, the inflammatory cells and fibroblasts are recruited from fracture hematoma with cellular proliferation and vascular ingrowth occur.
2. Repair or induction stage—pluripotential stem cells recruited to the area differentiate into bone forming cells and osteoid is laid down, which begins at periphery of fracture callus and progresses to inward within fracture callus and at conclusion of this stage a rubbery, minimally calcified woven bone is laid down directing to third stage of healing.
3. Remodeling stage—woven bone is laid down in the repair stage undergoes refinement. Cutting cones remove woven bone and osteoblasts lay down trabecular or lamellar bone in response to load on the bone over months and years and finally robust osseous tissue is formed to withstand the load.

Q.21 What are agents which interfere bone healing?
Ans. Non-steroidal anti-inflammatory drugs, steroids, tobacco.

Q.22 What are techniques used for preparation of allografts?
Ans. Fresh frozen allografts-though incorporate fast but there is great risk of disease transmission.

Freeze—dried allografts- less chances of transmission of diseases, but incorporate slowly, strength is inferior in torsion and bending.

Irradiation—leads to weakening of allografts in all axes.

Q.23 What are types of bone grafts?
Ans. Autografts—harvested from one site to another site, has good osteogenic property, especially in vascularised autogratfs.

Allografts—taken from one member of common species and transplanted into other, has weaker osteoinductive property but has good osteoconductive property.

Xenografts—taken from one species and transplanted into other species, not widely used, as stimulation of bone formation is not good.

Q.24 What are bone grafts substitute?
Ans. Bone derived substitutes—such as demineralised bone matrix (DBM)-Grafton-consists of bone from which the calcium hydroxyapatite salts have been removed provide source of osteoinductive proteins so possess osteoinductive properties though they are wreak and osteofil.

Synthetic (ceramic)—consists of mineral salts such as hydroxyapatite, calcium phosphate, calcium sulfate, or coralline-derived hydroxyapatite, where they can be in the form of paste, blocks, or tablets which are readily absorbed and possess osteoconductive properties.

Q.25 What are important applications of allografts?

Ans. Massive osteochondral grafts are used in limb saving surgery. They should be fresh with viable articular cartilage. Though they do not incorporate but unite with great success.

Q.26 What are types and indications of osteochondral allografts?

Ans.
- Osteochondral plug grafts are mainly used to repair damaged articular surfaces such as osteochondritis dissecans lesions.
- Unicondylar allografts—used at defects created by resection of benign tumors of knee—such as giant cell tumor, chondroblastoma but they are not useful for malignant tumors. Results are very good.
- Hemijoint allografts—used after resection of osteosarcoma, but difficult to get of ligamentous stability and implantation.
- Whole joint allografts—results are doubtful, difficult technique.

31 CHAPTER

Different Methods of Fracture Fixation

Q.1 What are shear, tension and compression forces?
Ans. The forces acting on the bone are either along the bone axis, i.e. axial force or perpendicular to axis, i.e. normal force. Or there may be parallel to axis, i.e. shear force. The normal and axial force may be either in the form of compression (pressing) or tension (pulling away).

Q.2 How does torsion affect?
Ans. Torsion is due to high shear and tension. Spiral fracture is initiated in shear force as bone is weaker parallel to axis and tension causes progression at 45° plane.

Q.3 Define stable and rigid fixation.
Ans. When there is no movement at fracture site in spite of joint movements, is stable fixation.
   When there is no deformation of any kind under load is rigid fixation.

Q.4 Why does butterfly fracture occur?
Ans. Combination of bending and axial compression leads to oblique, transverse and butterfly fractures.
   There is deformation due to bending force to concave side having compression force, convex side has tension force, axial, force causes further compression on concave side. Butterfly fragment is the result of all combinations of forces and change of oblique to transverse fracture.

Q.5 What are stress risers?
Ans. Stress is internal force resisting deformation and where the stress is higher than elsewhere is called as stress risers. They are maximum at discontinuity such as hole after drilling, sharp angles, grooves, weakening the bone and fractures may initiate at these points. Other examples are pathological fractures, refracture near callus or fracture at the end of rigid plating.

Q.6 What are implants made up of?
Ans. They are made up of 316 L stainless steel which is alloy of chromium (self regenerating protection of surface). Molybdenum (responsible for rigidity and elasticity-decreases rate of dissolution), nickel, manganese, silicon and carbon (responsible for strength).

Q.7 What is the advantage of titanium?
Ans. Titanium—less allergic, can be kept for long time in the body, less potential toxic ions
Stainless steel—economical, high elasticity

Q.8 What are the signs of implant failure?
Ans. Implant failures are:
Brittle—poor conductivity may cause this; head of screw may fail
Plastic—bending of implants permanently due to load beyond its yield strength and causes alignment of fracture
Fatigue—when load is more than endurance limit due to cyclic loading.

Q.9 What is pitch and lead of the screw?
Ans.
- Pitch—distance between adjacent threads
- Lead—distance screw travels on complete turn.

Q.10 What is the weakest point of screw?
Ans. The core diameter is the weakest point of screw.

Q.11 How do you decide ideal drill bit for bone?
Ans. Drill bit has cutting edge which is conical in shape and has two cutting edges which act as wedge. Ideal cutting edge angle should be 90° to 110°. Helix angle should be 240° for high clearance and rapid advance of drill.

Q.12 How does compression plate acts?
Ans. By compaction of fracture, reducing space between the fragments of bone, protecting blood supply as making the fragments more stable, and avoiding torsion or shear.

Q.13 What is static and dynamic compression in plating and intramedullary nailing?
Ans.
- Plating—when plate applied under tension produces static compression during rest or functioning limb.
  Dynamic compression—when plate transfers functional forces into compressive forces at fracture site.
- Nailing—when both interlocking screws are passed on both sides of fracture, it is static compression.
  Dynamic—when only one interlocking screw is passed through small fragment, it is called dynamic compression.

Q.14 How is compression achieved by plating?
Ans.
- By using self-compressing plates such as DCP
- Ironing devices—seen in tension band wiring, etc.

- Placing screws eccentrically in oval-shaped holes to have dynamic compression effect.

Q.15 What is ideal placement of screw?
Ans. Screw should not be placed through the fracture site and should not be closer than 1 cm of fracture site, otherwise fixation will become loose.

Q.16 How does lag screw work?
Ans. When compression is achieved between two bony fragments, producing pressure across fracture line by providing purchase of distal fragment by providing threads when screw is in distal fragment and turning in proximal fragment quite freely. Thus interfragmentary motion is reduced by increasing compression between fragments. Screws should be inserted through the centre and at right angles to fracture line. This is seen usually in fixation after cancellous screws.

Q.17 What is stress protection phenomenon?
Ans. There is osteopenia after healing of fracture and when screws remaining tight beneath the plate, called stress protection phenomenon.

Q.18 Why should implants should be removed?
Ans. In cases of infection, corrosion, mechanical problems to patient, refracture at the ends of plate, when stability is loosened and weakened. It is, after all, foreign material in the body so should be removed.

Q.19 What are ideal sites of plating?
Ans. They are—femur—anterolateral, tibia-lateral, humerus-posterior, radius-anterior in lower third and posterior in upper third, ulna-anterior.

Q.20 What are disadvantages of plating?
Ans. Longer incisions, wide exposure and wide stripping of periosteum so as to hamper blood supply, chances of refracture at ends of plate even after removal of plates, corrosion of plates more common, breakage and bending of plates.

Q.21 Where was Kuntscher nail used first and when?
Ans. For subtrochanteric fracture and in November, 1939, at Germany

Q.22 What are the advantages of reaming?
Ans. Widens medullary cavity for acceptance of wider intramedullary nail for better stability. More surface contact of nail and bone, insertion of nail becomes easier as it is postulated that nails should not be hammered with more power other-wise endosteal lining of bone will be damaged. By reaming endosteal debris comes out thru' fracture site and remains under periosteum and helps in healing of bone.

Q.23 What are disadvantages of reaming?

Ans. Weakens cortex if reamed too much, destroys medullary circulation, due to heat there is necrosis of bone, chances of infection are more, interference in endosteal callus.

Q.24 How do you calculate working length of nail?

Ans. Two points are to be marked where there is firm gripping by bone and this length is measured and this carries major load across fracture. This is effective length of nail.

Q.25 How do you remove broken nail in-united fracture of long bone?

Ans. First remove proximal broken nail by exposing the part. Then either distal part can be removed by hammering distally and getting out through distal end of bone by long punch or similar nail. A window is created distal to fracture site near the proximal end of broken nail and nail can be taken out manually by hook or any similar device. In case of broken interlocking nail, guidewire is bent at distal end like hook and thus nail may be removed.

Q.26 How broken nail is removed in ununited fracture?

Ans. Proximal nail can be removed easily. By exposing the proximal part. As fracture is not united, again a window is created at fracture site and through that distal end can be removed. Or the window is created distal to distal end of nail and hammered out proximally by similar nail or strong guidewire.

Q.27 What type of fixation is used for open fractures?

Ans. The aim is to stabilise the fracture and automatically soft tissues are also stabilised and they heal better.

So usually external fixators are used commonly either single plane or biplanar or thing fixators are used. It is better to avoid using plates and screw sin open fracture-except type I open fractures. Primary or delayed (after healing of wounds) intramedullary fixations (simple nails or interlocking nails) can be used in type I, II, and III open fractures. Or, initially, external fixators are used and after healing of the wound or skin intramedullary, fixations can be used safely.

Q.28 Which is to be repaired first in type IIIC open fractures—arterial repair or bone fixation?

Ans. Without fracture stability, one cannot repair arterial injury at all as movements of bones may disrupt the repair of vessels either by graft or shunting.

Q.29 What are known complications of bioabsorbale implants?

Ans. Sterile sinus tract formation, osteolysis, synovitis, and hypertrophic fibrous encapsulation.

Q.30 What are indications for external fixators?

Ans. *Indications*
- Stabilisation of severe open fractures
- Stabilisation of infected nonunions
- Correction of extremity malalignments and length discrepancies
- Initial stabilisation of soft tissue and bony disruption in polytrauma patients (damage control orthopaedics)
- Closed fracture with associated severe soft tissue injuries
- Severely comminuted diaphyseal and periarticular lesions
- Temporary transarticular stabilisation of severe soft tissue and ligamentous injuries, pelvic ring disruption, certain pediatric fractures, arthrodesis ligamentotaxis, osteotomies

Q.31 What are contraindications of external fixators?

Ans.
- Patient with compromised immune system
- Noncompliant patient who would not be able to ensure proper wire and pin care
- Pre-existing internal fixation that prohibits proper wire or pin placement
- Bone pathology precluding pin fixation.

Q.32 What are the types of external fixators?

Ans.
- They are ilizarov apparatus
- Taylor spatial frame
- Hoffman external fixation system
- Rail external fixator.

Q.33 What are the advantages of external fixation?

Ans.
- Less damage to blood supply of bone
- Minimal interference with soft-tissue cover
- Useful for stabilising open fractures
- Rigidity of fixation adjustable without surgery
- Good option in situations with risk of infection
- Requires less experience and surgical skills than standard ORIF
- Quite safe to use in cases of bone infection

Q.34 What are the disadvantages of external fixation?

Ans.
- Pin-penetrating the soft tissues
- Restricted joint motion
- Pin tract complications in long-lasting external fixation
- Cumbersome and not always well tolerated.

CHAPTER 32

Ilizarov Technique

Q.1 What is the Ilizarov method?
Ans. The Ilizarov method of transosseous osteosynthesis is the system of surgical and bloodless techniques for treating a great number of orthopaedic diseases and injuries both congenital and acquired.

Q.2 What is history of Ilizarov technique?
Ans. This system has been developed in Kurgan (Transurales, Russia) by an orthopaedic surgeon Gavriil Ilizarov and his team. In 1951, Gavriil Ilizarov offered his external fixator for fracture union that consisted of two metal rings round the bone and a pair tensioned wires in each ring that transfixed the bone and crossed inside it. In 1952, he published his first lengthening experience of 12.5 cm in the local newspaper. But the innovative surgeon had to fight for 20 years to make the medical society acknowledge and accept his method in the Union of Soviet Socialist Republics (USSR).

Q.3 How many techniques are there in Ilizarov method?
Ans. The system includes more than 800 techniques with the use of the Ilizarov external fixator for long bones, external minifixator for short bones, transpedicular external fixator for the spine and external systems that are used for pelvic orthopaedic conditions and skull pathology.

Q.4 Can this technique be used for height growth?
Ans. Yes, this is one of the first methods used for limb lengthening and height growth. In the recent years, the number of people who refer to orthopaedic surgeons with a wish to change their height has considerably grown. Since the middle of 1970s, more than 500 persons increased their stature at the Kurgan center due to indications to a lengthening procedure, and they are mainly patients with achondroplasia (dwarfs).

Q.5 How is it different from conventional orthopaedic techniques?
Ans. No treatment method in the history of reconstructive traumatology and orthopaedics has had such an evolutional development as the Ilizarov method of transosseous osteosynthesis. The method has been called universal as it can be used for almost entire range of skeletal pathology that requires reconstruction and bone reshaping. Nowadays, it has been used in associated fields of medicine

such as angiology, neurosurgery, oncology, stomatology, arthrology, veterinary, etc. in cases of congenital pathology or trauma sequelae. For 55% of those who are affected by orthopaedic pathology, it is the only method that can recover them or improve their condition. It is less traumatic as compared to other methods; and the intervention procedures are less in volume in case the patient needs a complex operation or repeated surgeries.

Q.6 On which principle, is modified ilizarov technique used in infected nonunions?

Ans. It is the principle of distraction-compression osteogenesis. The Ilizarov technique is a good salvage operation for infected nonunion of the femur. Limb salvage is preferable to prosthesis if the limb is viable.

Q.7 What are the indications of Ilizarov technique?

Ans. These are as follows: Simple and compound fractures of all long bones, comminuted fractures crush and degloving injuries, polytrauma, malunions, nonunions delayed unions, shortening, joint contractures, infections, fracture of spine with associated neurovascular and musculotendinous injuries, hand and foot trauma.

Q.8 What are the advantages of Ilizarav technique?

Ans. It is less traumatizing and almost noninvasive.

33 CHAPTER

Metabolic and Endocrine Disorders

Q.1 How many types of cartilages are there?
Ans. They are:
- Hyaline cartilage—at articular surfaces, growth plates, or physis
- Fibrocartilages—Menisci
- Elastic cartilages—at the ear

Q.2 What are zones of the growing epiphysis?
Ans. On the epiphyseal side, there are four zones:
1. Zone of growth
2. Zone of cartilage transformation
3. Zone of ossification
4. Metaphysis.

Q.3 What is osteoporosis?
Ans. Osteoporosis has been defined by the WHO as bone mineral density 2.5 standard deviation below mean of young. Bone mineral density signifies approximately 70% of bone strength.

Q.4 What is osteomalacia?
Ans. Osteomalacia is an osteopenic condition characterised by insufficient mineralisation of the bone matrix, where the onset may be at any age and may be due to chronic renal failure, vitamin D. Deficiency, and hypophosphatemic condition with pain in bones as a common symptom.

Q.5 What are risk factors for osteoporosis?
Ans. Female gender, increased age, estrogen deficiency, white race, low weight, low bodymass index, smoking history, previous history of fracture and family history of osteoporosis.

Q.6 What is the treatment of osteoporosis?
Ans.
- Supplementation of calcium of 1000 mg to 1500 mg daily
- Intake of vitamin D of 400 to 1000 IU daily
- Physical activity

- Taking of biphosphate such as risedronate, alendronate and etidronate
- Hormone replacement therapy such as traditional estrogen, to increase bone density.

Q.7 What is brown tumor?
Ans. Hyperparathyroidism, primary or secondary, causes typical changes in the bone, revealing several osteoclasts on the bone surface with resorption of bony trabeculae, which is of pericellular bone by osteocytes, increased woven bone and marrow replacement by dense-fibrous appearing tissue. During the course of hyperparathyroidism, there are radiolucent lesions of diaphysis of long bones, jaw, or skull, which appear brown due to recent or old haemorrhages with microscopic picture of numerous giant cells in the fibrous cellular stroma. These brown tumors regress dramatically as soon as hyperparathyroidism is controlled.

Q.8 What is cretinism?
Ans. It is a congenital hyperthyroidism giving picture of dwarfism with mental retardation, which is more common in females, with dry skin, scanty and coarse hair enlarged tongue, expressionless face, narrowed palpebral fissures, enlarged abdomen, umbilical hernia, and generalised lethargy. If treated properly, the prognosis is good for normal bone and mental development.

Q.9 What is rickets?
Ans. It is defined as inadequate calcification of bone matrix in immature skeleton.

Q.10 What are four causes rickets?
Ans. Vitamin-D deficiency, chronic renal insufficiency, renal tubular insufficiency, hypophosphatasia.

Q.11 What are clinical and radiological features of rickets?
Ans. *Clinical:* Muscular weakness, lethargy, protuberant abdomen, Craniotabes (enlarged forehead) and thickening of weight-bearing joints causing deformities at metaphyseal-epiphyseal junction.

Radiological: Thickened epiphyseal plate, brush border of metaphysis, flaring of metaphysis (trumpeting), thickening of osteochondral articulations of ribs causing rachitic rosary, diminished cortical density and coarse trabecular pattern, which is irregular and with wide space.

Q.12 What are the deformities caused by vitamin-D resistant rickets?
Ans.
- Genu varum or valgus
- Coxa vara
- Anterior bowing of femur
- Anterolateral bowing of tibia
- Protrusio acetabuli
- Kyphoscoliosis.

CHAPTER 34

The Art of Physiotherapy

Q.1 What is physical therapy?
Ans. This is the science used for rehabilitation of a patient after disease or injury.

So physical therapy is a branch, which is for diagnosis of dysfunction of movements, management to recover them, restore, maintain and promote optimal physical functions of the body, keeping fitness of the body, and prevention of such dysfunctions.

Q.2 What is occupational therapy?
Ans. Occupational therapy is therapeutic use of self-care, work, and play activities to increase independent function enhancing development and prevent disability.

Q.3 How does heat in physiotherapy help?
Ans. By increasing metabolism of the part, increasing extensibility of collagen leading to relieve pain and spasm.

Q.4 What are types of heat treatment?
Ans.
- Simple hot water bag or bottle—for conductive heating
- Wax bath—for conductive and latent heat
- Short wave diathermy—high frequency alternate electric current, there is agitation of molecules within the tissue and secondary heat is produced and the patient is relieved of pain and spasm. There are interferential heat therapy and microwave heat therapy.

Q.5 What are ultrasonics? What are the indications?
Ans. Ultrasound is frequency of sound wave which produces piezoelectric effect of voltage to ceramic disc with deep penetration.

Indicated for deep pain, for extension of scar, and due to tissue excitability, there is vasodilatation and thus pain is relieved.

Q.6 What is place of cryotherapy?
Ans. Ice is used to reduce blood loss, to reduce oedema and pain in recent injury and to reduce spasticity.

Q.7 How do you define electrotherapy?
Ans. When low frequency direct current applied either in the form of galvanic or ionization to relieve pain or for the treatment, it is called electrotherapy.

Q.8 What are the differences between galvanism and ionization?
Ans. *Galvanism:* Direct low frequency current of 1–2 mA when applied produces effect of analgesia under anode and counter-irritant effect under cathode, enhancing driving of specific ions such as histamine.

Ionization: This is process of driving ions into the tissue by an electric current, which is called iontophoresis or ionization. It has superficial effect.

Q.9 What is TNS?
Ans. This is transcutaneous nerve stimulation (TNS) based on Gate theory, which proposes both large and small diameter fibres synapse on common cells on spinal cord and stimulation of cord inhibits passage of sensory inflow to cortex and thus relief.

Q.10 What are different exercises?
Ans. *Passive exercises:* Movements done with assistance are passive exercises.

Active exercises: Movements done without any assistance are active exercises against gravity.

Assisted exercises: When therapist assists patient to do movements with active participation of the patient.

Q.11 What are resisted exercises?
Ans. They are:
- *Isometric exercises:* When movements due to plaster immobilization are not possible, then voluntary contractions are done, are also called static exercises. these help in maintaining bulk and tone of muscles.
- *Isotonic exercises:* These are used for developing of muscle power.
- *Mobilising exercises* are used for increasing movements of joint.

Q.12 On which principle do isokinetic exercises work?
Ans. Type I and II muscle fibres waste after disuse so, if regular, low repetition-high resistance followed by low resistance with repetition can build both types of muscle fibres.

CHAPTER 35

Orthoses, Braces, Splints

ORTHOSES

Q.1 What is orthotic device?
Ans. A device which provides correction or support for weak or imbalance muscles. An orthosis is force system that acts on body segments. Orthosis can be simple as a soft arch support in the shoe or complex as reciprocating gait orthosis, a brace that encompasses the pelvis and both hips, knees and ankles and the feet.

Q.2 What is function of orthosis?
Ans. Orthosis provides stability, overcomes weakness, relieves pain, and controls deformity.

Q.3 What are requirements of good prosthesis?
Ans. It should be enough strong, light in weight, simple, easy to apply and manipulation can be done.

Q.4 What is difference between terms brace, splint and orthotic?
Ans. *Brace:* This is layman's term for orthotic device, which is broadest term. Used for longer period for treatment of orthopaedic problems.
Splint is supportive device used for shorter period may after operation or injury.

Q.5 What is function of spinal orthotic devices?
Ans. They are supportive and corrective and for relieving pain, support weak muscles, unstable joints, immobilize vertebral column in functional position.

Q.6 What types of spinal orthoses are available?
Ans. *Supportive*—belts and corsets
Corrective—Milwaukee brace.

Q.7 What is orthosis used in neck region?
Ans. Cervical collar which is devised by Thomas, used from sheep skin. The principle is to maintain neck in physiological position, may be modified with shoulder strap.

Q.8 What are orthoses for lumbar spine?
Ans. They are braces, made up of metal frame encircling body such as Thomas, Taylors, Golwaith. There are corsets which are back support strengthened by few metallic bars and belts which are made of soft materials which are not stiff.

Q.9 What is Taylor's brace?

Ans. Devised by CF Taylor in 1863, rigid orthosis with metal frame having firm foundation on pelvis with pelvic corset. The posterolateral part is made of metal along with upright attached metals supporting each side of spinous processes acting like back levers, with horizontal bars extending laterally and anteriorly in thoracic region and infra-axillary. In addition abdominal and shoulder supports are provided.

Q.10 What are indications of Taylor's brace?

Ans. This is most useful in tuberculosis of spine at thoracolumbar region with advantages of limiting forward flexion, extension, and lateral flexion with rotation but with increased lumbosacral joint movements.

Q.11 What is Milwaukee's orthosis?

Ans. *Miwaukee's brace:* This is indicated in scoliosis, ankylosing spondylitis and tuberculosis of spine. Its main feature are made up of moulded leather corset with side two metal bars, being vertical bar posteriorly, passing upward with submental pad, with leather strap on posterior bar on convex side. Patient is advised to put cotton, keeping brace clean, skin has to be massaged frequently and patient should wear if continuously. There is complication of meralgia.

Q.12 What are supportive devices for the spine?

Ans. A support which stabilizes lumbosacral spine is called LS orthosis. LSO which may be rigid, bivalved or plastic. Spine support which is used for higher level of spine and used for thoracic spine is called, thoracic-lumbar-sacral orthosis. TLSO the support which is used for cervical spine is called CTLSO.

Q.13 What are corsets?

Ans. Corsets are spinal supports with posterior metal strip with object to restrict movements but not immobilizing completely.

Q.14 What are different corsets?

Ans. *Lumbosacral corset,* Usually 20–40 cm in width, extending up to thoracolumbar junction, fulcrum strap passing around pelvis. Metal strips may incorporated for more strength and rigidity. This does not interfere movements of hip and pelvis and posterior metal strips are moulded to curvature of spine.

Thoracolumbar corset, In addition to above, the width is more, has shoulder strap extending over scapula.

Q.15 What are lower limb orthoses?

Ans. These are meant for relieving weight bearing, pain and controlling deformity and movements.

There are many different types such as weight relieving used where low weight transmission is needed through bones, body weight supported on ring top weight transmission through metal bars, non weight relieving-ring merely locates upper end of side bar.

Q.16 What are supporting devices for lower limb?

Ans. Arch support for foot is called foot orthosis (FO) when support stabilizes foot and ankle then it is called AFO, when it is extended to knee it is then called KAFO, when extended to hip then is HKAFO. These orthoses may be solid, articulating or dynamic. Solid AFO does not allow ankle motion, articulating orthoses allows motion in one direction and preventing motion in another direction at various joints. There may be locks at knee and hip. In dynamic orthoses, there may be active motions against elastic resistance so that it come back to resting position.

Q.17 What different terminologies used for orthoses of lower limbs?

Ans. Hip, knee, ankle and foot are labeled as H, K, A and F respectively
- F. Free—for free movements
- A. Assisted—movements which are assisted
- R. Resisted—decrease some movements by external force
- S. stop—static inclusion
- H. Hold—to hold and maintain part in specific position.
- V. Variable—adjustable attachment
- L. Lock—for locking.

Q.18 What are supporting devices for upper limb?

Ans. WHO is wrist hand orthosis with specific function to perform. Above forearm, there is no universally accepted orthosis except shoulder—abduction splint.

Q.19 What is supporting device for ankle and foot?

Ans. Shoes with permeable flexion and extension or limiting theses movements with stirrups and heel sockets such as for varus foot—inside iron and outside T strap and for valgus outside iron bar with inside T strap.

Q.20 What locks are used for knee joint?

Ans. There is ring lock system at knee level with axis is eccentric preventing anterior edging during flexion and ring is pulled up to allow flexion of knee and pushed down in extension. There is another system of spring ring lock, which is used for automatic release of lock during extension. Swiss lock, which is used commonly now-a-days which is bar lock type system locks on extension by pulling on strap attached to posterior bar.

Q.21 Is there any nonlocking orthosis for knee joint?

Ans. This is used for cosmetic purpose for flail lower limb where the access of movement of joint posterior to flexion extension of knee.

Q.22 What are other attachments for knee?

Ans. They are anterior strap for mild flexion deformity of knee and posterior strap for genu recurvatum.

Q.23 What is orthosis used for equinus foot?

Ans. Toe-raising devices are used to abolish high stepping GAIT and tripping over uneven ground with back stop which controls planter flexion.

Q.24 How do you take care of orthoses?
Ans. These are avoiding dropping, pressure points are examined time to time, cleaning of dirt etc., oiling of joints of orthosis, and keep watch on heel and sole of shoes.

Q.25 What is caliper?
Ans. This is orthosis used for lower limb either on permanent or temporary basis to stabilize the weak limb, relieving weight bearing of weak limb, relieving pain, and restriction of joint movements.

Q.26 What is difference between surgical shoe and boot?
Ans. Surgical shoe is used for deformity when limited to forefoot up to midtarsal joints.

Boot is used for hind foot, with better grip and lacing extending up to toes for entry of foot.

Q.27 What are pressure points of cervical collar?
Ans. They are occiput and lower margin of mandible.

Q.28 How do you take measurements for collar?
Ans. Circumference of neck and distance between angle of jaw and clavicle.

Q.29 Where the collars are used best?
Ans. Collars are supposed to stabilize when the lesion is between C3 to C7.

Q.30 What are principles of collar?
Ans. They provide distraction between vertebrae and they try to shape the column but they cannot provide absolute immobilization.

Q.31 What is SOMI brace?
Ans. Sterno, occipito, mandibular immobilisation (SOMI) brace has same principle of four post-collar (occiput support, cupped plate for chin rest, back and chest support) but without back plate so that patient can lie down comfortably.

CORSETS

Q.1 What is corset?
Ans. Corset is an appliance, made of fabric with metal stiffness but without metal frame and this encircles the body.

Q.2 What is brace?
Ans. An appliance with metal frame and fabrics which supports body and encircles body is called brace.

Q.3 What is function of corset?

Ans. It gives corrective forces depending upon its efficiency when tightened.

Q.4 Upon which principle corset works?

Ans. Redistribution of weight bearing, shifting of centre of gravity towards spine by bringing closer abdominal wall to vertebral column.

But compression of abdominal wall tries to lengthen abdomen, and there is limitation for flexion of spine.

Q.5 What are different splints used for fingers?

Ans.
- *Mallet splint*—used for mallet finger by maintaining distal interphalangeal joint at full extension with permissible movements.
- *Frog splint*—used for distal phalanx mainly, by maintaining distal interphalangeal joint in full extension without any movements
- *Finger deviation splint*—used in rheumatoid arthritis for correction of deformity of proximal phalanx by passing wire from ulnar side to radial side of proximal phalanx
- *Armchair extension splint*—used for flexion contracture of fingers, has pad on volar aspect of metacarpal with spring wire at proximal phalanx and joined at pulp of finger.
- *Snake bangle*—used in rheumatoid arthritis to correct deformity has ulnar deviation effect, has thermoplastic material with stout spring wire.

Q.6 What are shoes used for knee deformities?

Ans.
- For genu valgum—wedge to inner border of soles and heels
- Mermaid splints—two gutter splints between legs of child with straps to correct deformity.

Q.7 What are walking aids?

Ans.
- *Walking frames*—used for elderly propel, in unstable people, and bedridden patients who are unable to use staircase. For this, it is necessary to have good muscle powers of flexors of fingers, dorsiflexors of hand and extensors of elbow.
- *Crutches: (a) Axillary crutches:* They are measured as: (i) Deduct 16 inches from height of patient; (ii) Measure distance from anterior axillary fold to edge of heel in supine position; (iii) Measure distance from anterior axillary fold to ground 4-6 inches lateral to foot, there is hand grip in 30° of elbow; *(b) Elbow crutches (Lotstrand crutches)*—Measured with 30° flexion at elbow, the tip of crutches is 6 inches lateral to tip of toes.
- Armband type—there should be 2 inches gap between top of arm and flexor crease of elbow.

Q.8 What are types of sticks used for lower limbs?
Ans. These are as stable as crutches but they are light in weight and easily operable They are: (A) Tripod and (B) Quadruped. Mainly, they are used for patients with neurological conditions.

Q.9 What are different crutch gaits?
Ans.
- *Swinging crutch gait:* This is for paraplegic patient when lower limbs are moved by trunk muscles due to weakness of muscles of lower limbs but body weight is taken by lower limbs. Body is swinging between the crutches.
- *Four point gait:* This is in unstable patients when whole or part of body weight is taken by foot the sequence is right crutch, left foot, left crutch and right foot
- *Two point crutch gait:* When the body weight taken by both feet is reduced when the balance of patient is good. The sequence is right crutch left foot simultaneously followed by left crutch and right foot.
- *Three point crutch gait:* Stronger limb takes body weight, affected limb takes partial weight or no weight as the affected limb is either weak or painful lower limb.

FUNCTIONAL CAST BRACING

Q.1 What are indications of functional cast bracing for knee joint?
Ans. *Indications are:*
- For fractures of distal one third of shaft of femur including supracondylar fracture
- For fracture of proximal one third of tibial shaft
- For comminuted fractures of condyles of femur and tibia
- Fracture of condyles of femur and tibia where open reduction with internal fixation are not indicated.

Q.2 What material is used for that?
Ans.
- Brace—an unicentric brace with two sizes bigger (one for adult and another for children) made up of aluminium with wings made up of thin malleable tin to enable to mould easily according to sizes of thigh and leg
- Alignment zig—to hold the brace and maintain in correct axis
- Stockinette—needed for initial compressive material and of appropriate size (apprx. 4 feet)
- Soft roll—to protect the skin over bony points which may be compressed by brace
- Plaster of paris bandages—good quality for fast setting and of 4" and 6" and 6 in numbers of each
- Screw driver and bar bender—for opening screws, to free hinges, and to bend brace according to required angle
- Spirit and antifungal powder—to clean the whole skin of thigh and leg and to prevent itching and infection.

Q.3 What are indications for ankle brace?
Ans.
- Fractures of middle and lower third of tibia
- Bilateral fracture of tibia
- Fractures in elderly people
- Compound fractures.

Q.4 What material is used for?
Ans.
- 4" 1- 4" × 4" plaster of paris bandages
- Stockinette
- Metallic joint incorporated in leather shoes
- Screw driver.

Q.5 When this cast should be removed?
Ans. An X-ray is taken to confirm about formation of callus, and then brace is removed and clinical tests for union are done such as no abnormal movements, no tenderness at fracture site.

Q.6 What are complications of brace?
Ans.
- Swelling of foot
- Angulation
- Loosening of nuts and screws
- Loosing or breaking of brace.

Q.7 What are indications for functional thigh sleeve?
Ans.
- Middle third and lower third fractures of shaft femur
- Postoperative of intramedullary nailing of shaft of femur.

Q.8 What are contraindications of functional thigh sleeve?
Ans.
- Wobbling fractures
- Upper third femoral shaft fractures
- Subtrochanteric fractures
- Supracondylar fracture of shaft of femur
- Bilateral fractures of shaft of femur
- Floating knee.

Q.9 What are indications of functional hip brace?
Ans.
- Subtrochanteric fractures
- Trochanteric fractures
- Upper third fracture of shaft of femur
- Postoperative of IM nailing.

Q.10 What are complications of hip brace?
Ans.
- Moderate oedema distal to brace
- Minor angulation deformity
- Loosening of brace
- Breaking of brace
- Loosening of nuts and bolts.

Q.11 What are indications of functional wrist brace?
Ans. Colles fracture, fracture of lower end of radius and ulna.

Q.12 What is aim of wrist brace?
Ans.
- Elbow flexion is allowed and restriction of extension to 30°
- It prevents supination and pronation
- It permits full palmer flexion and allows dorsiflexion of wrist to neutral
- Permits full range of finger movements.

Q.13 What are indications of Olecranon-condylar brace?
Ans.
- Fracture of both bones of forearm in position
- Isolated fracture of ulna
- In conservative treatment of fracture of both bones of forearm after closed reduction
- All operated cases of fracture of both bones of forearm such as Monteggia fracture dislocation. Galeazzi fracture, if there is no rigid fixation as an additional support.

Q.14 What are indications of elbow brace?
Ans.
- Intercondylar fractures of humerus
- Side sweep injuries of elbow
- Badly comminuted fracture of lower end of humerus which cannot be fixed
- Fractures of both bones of forearm after IM nailing. The brace should be ideally applied after formation of callus and fragments have become sticky.

CASTS

Q.1 What is function of casts?
Ans. Casts are used for immobilisation of limbs while treating fractures and after operations. They should not be used for paralytic limbs where sensory loss is there. They can be used for maintaining corrected position of limbs after manipulation casts may be made up of plaster of paris or plastic material. They are used for encouraging osteosynthesis, for promotion of healing tissues, and prevention of stiffness of joints.

These are external splints which are applied to fractures limb to provide adequate support till healing with permission of maximum function affected limb.

Q.2 What is method of application of casts?

Ans. Casts should not be applied directly to skin, some sorts of padding should be used. And they should be applied in circular manner with moulding to bony points. The casts are rigid. If there are open wounds, then windows should be made for inspection and dressing to avoid complications of gas gangrene and tetanus.

Q.3 What is composition of casting material?

Ans. Usually, the material used is plaster of Paris. The powder is embedded in the gauze, of different width. Fibre glass casting material has become more popular nowadays urethane material is embedded in knitted fiberglass rolls where the hardening is much quicker.

Q.4 What are another materials of casts?

Ans. Plaster of Paris, fiberglass, hexalite, thermoplastic.

Q.5 What guidelines for using casts?

Ans.
- Casts are to be used for immobilisation of fracture or fractured part
- Casts should be applied one joint below and one above
- Casts should not be used for reduction of fracture but used for maintaining the position
- When casts are dried, then they become loose and fractures may get displaced.
- Cases should be applied in such a way that they should not be too tight to hamper neurological or vascular conditions of the limb
- Additional pins may be used in the casts to stabilize the fractures.

Q.6 When casts should be applied?

Ans.
- Functional casts should not applied immediately after injury, but applied after correction of angulation or rotational deformity
- Minor movements at fracture site should not be painful
- Deformity should get disappeared, once it has been corrected
- There should be reasonable resistance to telescoping
- Shortening should not exceed more than 1/4th inch for tibia and ½th inch for femur.

Q.7 What are contraindications for casts?

Ans. They should not be applied in:
- Mentally retarded patients
- Uncooperative patients
- Patients with peripheral vascular diseases and neuropathy
- Skin loss or any skin problems.

Protheses

Q.1 What is pylon?
Ans. This is temporary prothesis used at earlier stage and immediately after operation, which provides central core of limb around which prosthesis is built and gives best moral and psychological support to patient.

Q.2 What type of prosthesis is used for disarticulation of hip?
Ans. This is turning table type prosthesis, which has socket embracing whole pelvis above iliac crest. providing suspension, where the weight is taken by ischial tuberosity and rest of socket is like above knee prosthesis.

Q.3 What is PTB prosthesis?
Ans. This is patellar tendon bearing (PTB) type of prosthesis where there is total contact type of fitting socket, based on the principle of maximum weight is taken by patellar ligament and its expansion. All stresses in all directions are taken on knee so does not need knee support.

Q.4 What is SACH foot?
Ans. Solid-Ankle Cushion Heel (SACH) has components as follows: Wooden keel with 2-mm bonded canvas, high density of rubber on dorsum, low density rubber at toes on planter aspect with variable density rubber heel.
    This has got solid ankle cushion heel foot, without any ankle joint but ankle movements are provided by compression of wedge shaped rubber heel. This is simple and smooth transition from heel contact to toe off.

Q.5 What are Syme's appliances?
Ans. This is closed or open socket type:
- *Open type:* It has blocked leather socket which is open at the bottom but closed for 10 cm at top to give tibial support
- *Closed type:* This does not have too bulbous stump end and socket is closed.

Q.6 What is Jaipur foot?
Ans. This is devised by Professor Dr PK Sethi of Jaipur. This can be used for bare foot walking also which is made up from vulcanized rubber and mRC with two wooden blocks instead of single wooden keel. This has got facility of toe break which allows inversion and eversion of foot which has broad based and micro cellular rubber which helps in bare foot walking. This is most economical and cost effective.

37
CHAPTER

Diagnostic Radiology

Q.1 What are common radiographic views for shoulder problems?
Ans. Usually, anteroposterior views are commonly taken but some time in neutral position view is also taken in external or internal rotation. Axillary view is also important to assess position of humeral head in the glenoid cavity.

Q.2 What are types of dislocations of shoulder? Which is more common?
Ans. Anterior dislocation is much more common—incidence about 95%, than posterior dislocation which is just 5%.

Q.3 How do you differentiate between anterior and posterior dislocations?
Ans. They are best differentiated by axillary view. X-ray beam is directed from inferior position through the axilla to superior plate.

Q.4 How do define Bankart's lesion?
Ans. A Bankart's lesion is an avulsion of anterior capsular structures with fragment of bone. This lesion most common in recurrent dislocation of shoulder and best seen in axillary view.

Q.5 What is a Hill-Sachs lesion?
Ans. This is defect in the posterolateral aspect of humeral head which occurs with anterior dislocation of shoulder when posterior superior surface of humeral head impinges on anteroinferior portion of glenoid. This is easily visualised by anteroposterior view of shoulder with arm in full internal rotation.

Q.6 What is role of radiology in impingement syndrome?
Ans. The supraspinatus outlet view is helpful in evaluating this syndrome. Patient is put as in lateral scapular. X-ray and tube is angled inferiorly at 10° where it is seen the morphology of acromion for the treatment of this syndrome.

Q.7 What is radiological appearance in acromioclavicular dislocation?
Ans. In this dislocation, there is disruption of coracoclavicular and acromioclavicular ligaments and space is widened between clavicle and coracoid where the clavicle is displaced superiorly in comparison with acromion when there is complete dissociation of acromioclavicular joint anteroposterior view is taken with 10–15 pounds of weight in each arm for better visualization.

Diagnostic Radiology   **149**

Q.8 How do you evaluate radiologically elbow symptoms?
Ans. Anteroposterior and lateral view are sufficient most of the time. Fractures of radial head, loose bodies in olecranon fossa, or anteriorly in the anterior joint, osteochondritis dissecans seen as irregularities along with capitellum can be diagnosed with these routine views.

Q.9 What is pathological fracture?
Ans. A pathological fracture occurs when the bone is weakened by infection, neoplasm, or metabolic bone disease. But common causes are benign tumors of bone, osteomyelitis and tuberculosis of bone.

Q.10 What is radiological picture of acute osteomyelitis?
Ans. In early stage, there is blurring or obliteration of soft tissue fat planes, followed by intramedullary destruction and then there is cortical destruction, endosteal scalloping and periosteal reaction, but the radiological changes take some time to show on plain X-ray say 10–14 days but by this time, the disease has been spread over.

Q.11 What is study of choice in suspected osteomyelitis?
Ans. As usual plain X-rays are taken. Three phase bone scan is good for diagnosis of acute osteomyelitis at early stage by showing increased activity on perfusion, blood pool, and delayed images in the area of bony involvement are compatible to osteomyelitis. MRI also can give good idea at early stage, which shows oedema of marrow, early cortical destruction and soft tissue abscess clinch to diagnosis of osteomyelitis.

Q.12 What is charcot joint?
Ans. This is also called neuropathic joint, occurring in patients with neurologic neuropathy secondary to diabetes mellitus, syphilis, paraplegia, leprosy, and other peripheral neuropathies. Patients loose sensations of pain and proprioception but motion is maintained. Subtle fractures occur with significant degenerative changes. X-ray shows joint destruction, with bony debris from fractures, loose bodies, and disorganization of joint occurs with subluxation or dislocation.

Q.13 What is Salter Harris classification for epiphyseal fractures?
Ans. They are classified as:
- *Type I:* Separation of epiphyseal plate with fracture line is in the cartilage which is not visible on plain X-ray.
- *Type II:* In this common injury, there is fragment of metaphysis along with epiphyseal plate fracture
- *Type III:* Fracture runs through the epiphysis and growth plate.
- *Type IV:* A vertical fracture line through epiphysis and growth plate extending into metaphysis may be followed by arrest of growth, joint deformities
- *Type V:* Crushing injury to epiphyseal plate which results in shortening or angulation of bone due to premature closure of epiphyseal plate.

Q.14 How a patient of cervical spine trauma is evaluated with which initial film?

Ans. The first film to get is a cross table lateral view where all cervical seven vertebrae have to be visualized. Cervicothoracic junction is common site of traumatic injury.

Q.15 In normal, cross-table lateral view is further imaging necessary?

Ans. Yes, minimal evaluation of cervical spine must include a lateral view, an anteroposterior view and view of odontoid. Some important injuries may not be visible on lateral views.

Q.16 What are radiological studies to be done for evaluating hip disease?

Ans. Anteroposterior of pelvis should be taken to study of both hips as comparative study. This view gives idea about pelvic bones, lower portion of spine, sacroiliac joints, pubic symphysis. Joint changes may indicate about ankylosing spondylitis and rheumatoid arthritis. Bone destructions after secondaries or multiple myeloma are best seen in pelvic bones and fractures of ring of pelvis can be easily seen by comparing other iliac crest, pubic and ishial rami.

Q.17 What lines and angle are useful in evaluating pediatric hip for developing dysplasia?

Ans.
- *Hilgenreiner line:* Line connecting the triradiate cartilage.
- *Perkins:* Perpendicular to Hilgenreiner's line through lateral acetabular rim
- *Shenton:* Arc formed by the inferior surface of the superior pubic ramus and medial surface of the femoral metaphysis.
- *Acetabular angle:* Angle between the line drawn from superolateral ossified acetabular edge to triradiate cartilage and Hilgenreiner's line <30° suggests dysplasia.

Q.18 What are common sites of fatigue fractures?

Ans. They are tibial shaft, mid-fibula, pubic ramus, metatarsals, calcaneum, pars interarticularis.

Q.19 What are types of stress fractures?

Ans. They are divided into two categories:
1. *Fatigue fractures*, which occur due to repetitive prolonged stress on normal bone
2. *Insufficiency fractures*, occurring after normal stress on abnormal bone.

Q.20 What are predisposing conditions causing to insufficiency fractures?

Ans. They are osteomalacia, Paget's disease, osteoporosis, fibrous dysplasia, hyperparathyroidism, and in addition to radiation to bones.

Q.21 How stress fracture look radiologically?

Ans. Usually, they are seen as transverse fractures in the shaft of bone. Such as metatarsal stress fracture are seen slight, thin, radiolucent line. But they are better seen on larger bones such as tibia or femur. Sometimes fracture lines are not seen but healing of bone with new bone formation may be seen in the form of callus which may be abundant in metatarsals and may be minimal in tibia or femur.

Q.22 What is avascular necrosis?
Ans. This is also known as osteonecrosis which is bone death followed by vascular insufficiency. The vessels may be damaged directly by trauma or occluded by emboli or elevated marrow pressure. The common sites are hips, shoulders, medial femoral condyle and talus and scaphoid.

Q.23 What are causative factors of AVN?
Ans. They are overuse and prolonged use of steroids, alcohol, sickle cell disease, emboli, Caisson's disease, radiation therapy, Gaucher's disease, lupus erythematosus, any congenital problem, pancreatitis and fractures.

Q.24 What are radiological features of osteonecrosis?
Ans. In early stages, there are hardly any diagnostic features on plain X-ray.
- Bone scan is only helpful at this stage.
- But at later stage, there are changes like: (1) Bone cysts with sclerotic margins; (2) Subchondral collapse with or without flattening of articular surface; (3) Narrowing of joint space; (4) Other degenerative signs, which may be minimal but are progressive, which are joint space narrowing, osteophytes, subchondral cysts and subchondral sclerosis.

Q.25 What are radiological features of slow growing or benign lesion of bone?
Ans. These are:
- Preservation of cortical margin
- Well demarcated boundary of lesion
- Sclerotic margin
- Solid and uninterrupted periosteal reaction
- Little or no soft tissue mass except in osteomyelitis.

Q.26 What are radiological features of malignant lesions?
Ans.
- Cortical erosion and destruction
- Irregular periosteal reaction with sunburst onion peeling or Codman's triangle
- Absence of sclerotic margin
- Associated soft tissue mass
- Boundaries of lesion are not clear and spread of lesion in the adjacent soft tissue and bone.

Q.27 How do you describe Codman's triangle?
Ans. This is found with infraction or tumor which is mainly radiological feature. When tumor or infection starts elevating periosteum and gap is created between periosteum and bone, there is new bone formation in this gap, which is

triangular in shape on plain X-ray and this is what Codman's triangle, which was first described by Rubbert in 1914, denoting soft tissue extension. Though it is considered as feature of malignant tumor but can be seen in disorders where the periosteum is elevated either by benign or malignant tumor or infection.

Q.28 What is Jones fracture?

Ans. A Jones fracture is a transverse fracture of fifth metatarsal at proximal part, which is located 1.5-2 cm distal to tip of metatarsal usually stress fracture. It has to differentiated from styloid process fracture of metatarsal which occurs at metaphysis, which is seen on oblique view of foot. Normal apophysis in children may not be fused and may give appearance of fracture.

Q.29 What is second fracture?

Ans. Second fracture is an avulsion fracture of capsular ligament on lateral side of tibia, which is best seen on anteroposterior view of knee joint. It is highly suggestive of an anterior cruciate ligament tear as both are commonly associated.

Q.30 What views are taken for evaluation of ankle injuries?

Ans. Proper assessment of ankle mortise is very important in ankle injuries. So usual anteroposterior and lateral views are taken with oblique view with approximately in 20-30° in internal rotation of ankle can give better picture of ankle mortise. The level of medial and lateral malleolus, which are on same plane in mortise view, can give clue about congruity of talus as it sits adjacent to medial and lateral malleolus and tibial plafond.

Q.31 Which abnormalities of talus are seen on radiographs?

Ans. Fracture of talar dome or neck may be seen on usual ankle X-rays. Where dome fracture are related to inversion or eversion injuries which occur at superolateral or superomedial portion of talar dome, which are seen as small, separated fracture. It is some times necessary to take anteroposterior view in full plantar flexion.

Q.32 What are radiological features of inversion injury of ankle?

Ans. Ligaments of ankle joint are very strong. So with inversion injuries of foot and ankle, avulsive forces affect lateral structures and with compressive forces medial structures are affected. Ligamentous injuries are not visible on X-ray, but if there is fracture which is usually transverse with avulsion of ligaments. Fracture can be visualized on anteroposterior and oblique views. Medial inversion injury may show oblique fracture of medial malleolus, but in general oblique fractures are due to compressive forces.

Q.33 How eversion injury may project on X-ray?

Ans. With eversion injuries, avulsive forces affect on medial structures and compression forces act on lateral structures. Rotation of ankle at the time of injury play get role such as sprain or avulsion of medial spring ligament may occur which is not seen on X-ray. But if fracture occurs, then it is transverse fracture of medial malleolus below the level of ankle mortise. Lateral injuries may cause oblique or spiral fracture of lateral malleolus with rupture of syndesmosis with or without injury to tibiofibular ligament with or without fracture of fibula.

Q.34 What radiographic abnormality is seen in patients with peroneal tendon dislocations?
Ans. Peroneal tendon dislocations cause avulsion of osteocartilaginous attachment of peroneal tendon sheath to fibula resulting in small avulsion fracture of posterolateral corner of distal fibula, indicating hallmark of radiological appearance of peroneal tendon subluxation.

Q.35 How do you evaluate radiologically knee pathology?
Ans. The usual anteroposterior and lateral views of knee can give much idea about metaphyseal bone of femur, fibula, joint surfaces and surrounding soft tissue. A special, tunnel view of knee can give idea about intercondylar notch and loose bodies which are not seen in usual anteroposterior views. This view can show osteochondritis dissecans of medial or lateral femoral condyle. A sunrise Hughston view shows subluxation or dislocations of patella from trochlear groove.

Q.36 What are important radiological examinations in patients of rheumatoid disease?
Ans. An anteroposterior view of hand shows many joints of wrist and phalanges as rheumatoid arthritis affect as entire wrist, metacarpophalangeal joints. Osteoarthritis usually affects interphalangeal joints of fingers and first carpometacarpal joint. In erosive OA there is destruction of interphalangeal joint, severe erosions and with sublimations.

Erosions in gout may project as overhanging margins.

X-ray of patients with calcium pyrophostate dihydrate deposition disease may show subchondral cysts, interarticular soft tissue calcification mostly at radial styloid and triangular fibrocartilage.

Q.37 Is it normal to see anterior or posterior pad of fat in lateral X-ray of flexed elbow?
Ans. The anterior pad of fat appears as lucid stripe which is parallel to anterior margin of supracondylar region and if this assumes sail-shaped configuration, then the elbow capsule is distended indicating recent trauma causing hemarthrosis.

Posterior pad of fat is not seen in lateral view but if visualized, indicates distension of elbow capsule may be due to hemarthrosis due to undisplaced fracture of radial head.

CHAPTER 38

Computed Tomography and Magnetic Resonance Imaging

Q.1 Which modality of imaging is good for visualisation of complex hip fracture?

Ans. Computed tomography (CT) gives best knowledge about extent of fracture, displacement and fracture fragments within joint space. Three-dimensional CT gives still better idea about anatomical depth.

Q.2 How do you diagnose fracture of sacrum in a better way?

Ans. CT is better than plain X-ray, which may not give idea for several days.

Q.3 How sternoclavicular dislocation is best defined?

Ans. CT is better and rapid way to diagnose this dislocation with more accuracy than plain X-ray even mediastinal trauma may be better defined with CT.

Q.4 What is the best way to evaluate Lisfranc fracture?

Ans. Plain X-ray followed by CT in coronal plane.

Q.5 How do you diagnose tarsal coalition in a better way?

Ans. CT is best way to diagnose and define bony coalition with identification of facets. Even fibrous coalition may project as irregular and roughened cortical surfaces. But magnetic resonance imaging (MRI) is better method to define bony coalition as it is multiplanar.

Q.6 Which is the sensitive method of imaging to evaluate tear in glenoid labrum?

Ans. CT arthrography or MR arthrography are most sensitive methods to detect these tears. Then routine MRI sensitivity may be about 95%.

Q.7 Which is the best way to evaluate suspected lumbar herniated disc?

Ans. CT scan gives better image for suspected herniated disc and any cortical changes of vertebra. MRI gives better idea about degenerative disc disease and can give direct sagittal image.

Q.8 How do you evaluate and with what method, low back pain after disc removal?

Ans. MRI gives better idea about epidural scar after operation and spinal canal stenosis and arachnoiditis than CT scan.

Q.9 How do you diagnose pseudarthrosis after operation of fusion of spine?
Ans. With CT scan, one can get better idea about this rather than MRI.

Q.10 What are two types of spondylolisthesis?
Ans. They are: (a) Lytic and (b) Degenerative.
- Lytic type is due to bilateral fractures or congenital defects in pars interarticularis and resulting in posterior displacement of superior vertebra over inferior vertebra.
- Degenerative type is due to degenerative erosions of superior facet of inferior vertebral body allowing forward movement of the inferior facet of superior body leading to spondylolisthesis. CT scan can also give idea about degree of displacement and defects in pars interarticularis.

Q.11 Which imaging method is better choice to evaluate soft tissue mass in the extremity?
Ans. MRI is good for soft tissue differentiation and CT scan is better for bony details.

Q.12 What pulse sequences are most commonly used in MRI of musculoskeletal system?
Ans. Conventional spin-echo T1-weighted, proton density, T12-weighted images are used often. Gradient-echo and inversion recovery short tau inversion recovery (STIR) images are also common.

Q.13 What are true contraindications to MRI?
Ans. Patients with internal cardiac pacemaker, brain aneurysm clip, metallic foreign body in the eye, cochlear implant, surgically implanted drug infusion pumps, neurostimulators, or bone growth stimulators, should not undergo MRI examination.

Q.14 Can a patient with orthopaedic implants under MRI?
Ans. Orthopaedic plates, nails or screws do not cause significant distortion of MRI signals. They may be better visualised with MRI. But prosthesis of hip or knee may cause some distortion adjacent to implant but normal hip or knee can be visualised by MRI, if needed.

Q.15 What is normal appearance of meniscus on MRI?
Ans. The intact meniscus demonstrates homogeneous low signal intensity on pulse sequences. The accuracy evaluation of meniscal tears on MRI is to the tune of 90%.

Q.16 How grading of abnormal signal intensity is done to classify meniscal tears?
Ans. There are three grades:
1. Early mucinous degeneration of meniscus shown as globular foci in normal volunteers and are of no clinical significance.

2. Linear horizontal area of increased signal intensity, not extending to articular surface but contacting capsular margin.
3. Torn meniscus is seen as abnormal signal intensity extending to articular surface.

In Grade I and II, menisci are seen normal arthroscopically but Grade III is seen clearly as torn meniscus by arthroscope.

Q.17 How do you define discoid meniscus of knee? What are its complications?

Ans. This is dysplastic meniscus which has got broad and disk-like configuration. Lateral discoid meniscus is more common. The complications are of tears and cysts.

Q.18 How do you diagnose ACL tear on MRI?

Ans. A complete tear is nonvisualization of normal low-signal intensity anterior cruciate ligament (ACL). In acute tear MRI shows effusion in the joint space and edematous pseudomass. Most of the tears are mid-to-proximal portion of ACL.

Q.19 What are pathological findings shown on MRI in cases of lateral patellar dislocation?

Ans. Torn medial retinaculum, lateral subluxation of patella, osteochondral fracture of patella, joint effusion and dysplastic patella, shallow or hypoplastic femoral groove, impaction bone bruise of lateral femoral condyle.

Q.20 What is classical location of osteochondritis dissecans of knee?

Ans. Osteochondritis dissecans of knee is located classically in non-weight bearing lateral aspect of medial femoral condyle, usually seen in males with usual history of trauma and best seen on MRI.

Q.21 What are other injuries associated with tear of medial collateral ligament of knee?

Ans. It may be associated with tears of ACL, medial meniscus, medial or posterior capsular tear, and impaction injury of lateral femoral condyle and lateral tibial plateau, can be well-visualised by MRI.

Q.22 What is best imaging method for evaluation of avascular necrosis of femoral head at early stage?

Ans. MRI is best choice to study and differentiate between avascular necrosis (AVN) from non-AVN head with sensitivity upto 97%. In addition nuclear scintigraphy with technetium-99-m labeled phosphate compounds also gives good idea about AVN at early stage. As early diagnosis can lead to successful result by efficient treatment.

Q.23 What is the best way to diagnose undisplaced fracture neck of femur when plain X-ray is normal?

Ans. MRI is most useful for this as MRI is able to depict the morphology of undisplaced fracture more accurately than any other imaging study.

Q.24 Which is nerve compressed in tarsal tunnel syndrome?
Ans. Posterior tibial nerve is entrapped and compressed in tarsal tunnel syndrome which is best studied by MRI, ganglion, neuroma, cysts, lipoma, varicose veins, tenosynovitis may be probable causes of compression.

Q.25 What is the common site for rupture of tendo-Achilles?
Ans. It is 2-6 cm above its insertion or os calcis which may be missed on clinical examination but can be well visualised on MRI.

Q.26 Which tendon is commonly ruptured in flat foot?
Ans. It is posterior tibial tendon which can be diagnosed by MRI (partial or complete).

Q.27 Which muscles form rotator cuff?
Ans. These are supraspinatus, infraspinatus, teres minor (SIT) and subscapularis.

Q.28 Which tendon is ruptured first?
Ans. Usually, it starts along with anterolateral edge of supraspinatus at its insertion into greater tuberosity of humerus.

Q.29 What are important abnormal anatomical etiologies of impingement syndrome seen on MRI?
Ans. They are—subacromial osteophytes, abnormality of shape and slope of acromion process, abnormality of morphology of acromioclavicular joint can be well visualised on MRI.

Q.30 How are abnormal tendons of rotator cuff classified on MRI?
Ans. There are three grades:
- Grade I—tendinitis—normal morphology with high signal intensity on T1-weighted images and normal low signals intensity on T2-weighted images.
- Grade II—partial thickness tears on either side of articular or bursal surface of the tendon and are seen as high signal intensity lesions on T2-weighted images.
- Grade III—lesions are full thickness tears that slow a high signal intensity gap in the tendon on T2-weighted images.

Q.31 What is the common appearance of AVN of scaphoid bone on MRI?
Ans. Low signal intensity on both T1 and T2 weighted images with occasional increased signals may be noted due to edema of marrow and fluid accumulation.

Q.32 Which carpal bone is affected in Kienbock's disease?
Ans. It is AVN of lunate bone which best seen on MRI.

Q.33 What is best imaging method to study pathology of cervical or thoracic spine?

Ans. MRI is best method to study pathology of cervical or thoracic spine about extradural lesions, intervertebral disc lesions, intradural pathology, and spinal cord pathology.

Q.34 How do you diagnose spinal infection?

Ans. MRI is best choice to get idea about discitis, osteomyelitis of vertebra, epidural abscess.

Q.35 Which method is good for study of bone marrow?

Ans. MRI directly images bone marrow and highly sensitive for finding out early secondaries, lymphoma, myeloma.

Q.36 Can MRI differentiate between benign and malignant lesion?

Ans. No, no specific signals intensity are seen for differentiating between benign and malignant lesions.

Q.37 Which imaging method is first choice to evaluate brachial plexus injury?

Ans. MRI is best choice.

CHAPTER 39

Nuclear Medicine

Q.1 What is nuclear medicine?
Ans. This is the study of images demonstrating physiology of organs after administering radiolabeled drugs, which is extract of specific organs where observation is made about function of organ through recorded images of activity distribution.

Q.2 What is a bone scan?
Ans. A bone scan uses physiological marker to detect abnormalities of bone metabolism, may be of whole body or may be limited to specific region by radiolabeled phosphorus-based compound.

Q.3 What is three-phase bone scan?
Ans. This consists of:
- Radionuclide angiogram centred over area of affection and done during injection
- Blood pool images of that area are taken after injection
- Delayed images may be taken after 2-3 hours after injection.

Q.4 What are the scintigraphic features of osteomyelitis?
Ans. In presence of osteomyelitis, angiogram will show focally increased blood flow. Blood pool and delayed images also show increased activity, which is more focal on delayed scan.

Q.5 What are three bones that are studied more effectively with nuclear medicine than with plain X-ray in trauma?
Ans. Sternum, scapula, and sacrum

Q.6 What does the H-shaped pattern of increased activity in the sacrum indicate?
Ans. Bilateral, linear and transverse increased activities are characteristic of sacral insufficiency fractures. Osteoporosis is main underlying cause.

Q.7 What is Legg-Calvé-Perthes disease?
Ans. This is the disease of capital femoral epiphysis showing avascular necrosis, occurring between ages of 5-7 years (usually), more common in males, In early

stage, radionuclide scanning is used to evaluate the vascular supply of femoral head and scintigraphic studies will show cold area in the proximal epiphysis even with early stage of disease.

Q.8 What are other common sites of avascular necrosis?

Ans. They are lunate, scaphoid, body of talus, and knee.

Q.9 What are scintigraphic features of osteitis pubis?

Ans. Bilateral increased activity at pubic rami by symphysis is demonstrated with osteitis pubis.

Q.10 How do you define reflex sympathetic dystrophy syndrome (RSDS)?

Ans. This is a symptom complex consisting of pain, vasomotor instability, swelling and dystrophc skin changes with history of trauma ore injury is self-limited syndrome but may become chronic and irreversible usually involving the upper extremity.

Q.11 What are scintigraphic features of RSDS?

Ans. Three-phase bone scan shows increased blood flow to the affected limb with increased activity on blood pool images, and on delayed images increased juxta-articular is noted around all-joint activity.

Q.12 What are scintigraphic features of loosening of prosthesis?

Ans. Bone scan will show increased activity of loosened prosthesis usually at distal end of femoral component or around the shaft of femur or acetabulum, not very reliable within 9–12 months after surgery.

Q.13 What are primary cancers which metastasize to bone?

Ans. They are breast cancer, lung cancer, prostate cancer, lymphoma and renal cell carcinoma, bone scans are quite sensitive and will show areas of abnormal increased activity.

Q.14 What is superscan?

Ans. Due to lack of renal activity and soft tissue activity, diffuse increased uptake is noted throughout skeleton, metastatic disease may be the most common cause usually from prostate and breast, in addition, they may be from fibrous dysplasia and Paget's disease, osteomalacia, hyperparathyroidism.

40
CHAPTER

Ward Rounds, Suture Materials, Methods of Sterilisation and OT Techniques

WARD ROUNDS: SOME PRACTICAL TIPS

Q.1 What are the contraindications of negative suction drainage?
Ans. At donor site of bone grafts, tear in dura mater, and when suction irrigation is done.

Q.2 Who used Plaster of Paris bandages for first time?
Ans. Antonius Mathijsen used Plaster of paris for the first time.
    When Henry III visited Paris in 1254, he was admired the smoother whiteness of walls and popularised use of plaster of Paris for walls of England.

Q.3 How many squares should be there per square cm in POP bandages?
Ans. They should be 16.

Q.4 What are various sites for skeletal traction?
Ans.
- Head—skull traction for fracture dislocation of cervical spine
- Olecranon—used to give Dunlop traction for comminuted supracondylar fractures of humerus
- Upper end of tibia—usually used for fractures of shaft of femur, intertrochanteric fractures, subtrochanteric fractures
- Lower end of femur—fractures of shaft of femur
- Ribs—for fractures of ribs with lung complications
- Calcaneum—for reduction of tibial shaft fractures during interlocking nailing.

Q.5 What is Charnley's traction unit?
Ans. This is used for ipsilateral fractures of lower limbs where pin is passed in upper tibia which is incorporated in below knee POP cast.

Q.6 What are fixed and balanced traction?
Ans. *Fixed traction:* Where counter traction is obtained by applying force against a fixed point to attachments of muscles in spasm.

Balanced traction: Where traction is balanced by counter traction through weight of body against gravity.

Q.7 What is role of traction?
Ans. Traction overcomes deforming force, relieves spasm, pain, controls movements of affected part.

Q.8 What are contraindications of skin traction?
Ans. Where skin has abrasions, lacerations, dermatitis, and impaired circulation.

Q.9 What is function of Bohler's stirrup?
Ans. This allows direction of traction to be varied without turning the pin in the bone.

Q.10 What are the complications of keeping upper tibial tracion pin for long time?
Ans. Infection at site of insertion such as osteomyelitis and sometimes anterior portion to pin may become sequestrated, predisposes stiffness of knee from fibrosis of extensor mechanism of knee, pin may become loose and may be turning by itself.

Q.11 How do you insert Steinmann's pin in upper end of tibia?
Ans. Under local anaesthesia and aseptic precautions, part is prepared, (painted and draped). While assistant holding limb in lateral rotation, small skin incision is taken at site of insertion of pin to avoid local skin necrosis, with chuck in which pin is inserted and fixed. By screwing movements, pin is inserted from medial side of cortex just 2.5 cm below and medially to tibial tuberosity, till it reaches to opposite cortex and nick is taken on opposite skin and pin is advanced further to desired length for application of stirrup leaving equal distance on both sides. And then bolts of stirrup are tightened. Wound is closed and roller gauze or dressing is applied soaked with tincture benzoin.

Q.12 How do you correct fixed flexion deformity of hip?
Ans. By Agnes Hunt traction.

Q.13 What are water resistant POP casts?
Ans. When melamine synthetic resin used with plaster of Paris form water resistant cast.

Q.14 How do you measure length of Thomas' splint?
Ans. In Thomas' splint for lower limbs which is called Thomas bed knee splint, the bars are of unequal lengths to accommodate and the ring is slanting position. Inner bar is short which is on medial side and outer bar is longer is on lateral side. The length is measured from groin to heel and 8-9 inches are added for traction purpose.

Thomas splint for upper limb: Both bars are equal in lengths and measured from axial to tip of fingers and 5-6 inches are added to get correct length and the ring is straight.

STERILISATION

Q.1 What is pressure and temperature used in autoclaves?
Ans. *Temperature:* 121°C is achieved by pressure 1516/sq. inch for 20 minutes but for gloved, it should be 109°C under pressure of 516/sq. inch for 30 minutes.

Q.2 What are methods of sterilisation with what agents?
Ans.
  A. *Physical method:*
     Dry heat   By way of flaming
     Moist heat   By way of boiling for 25-30 minutes
  B. *Radiation:*
     Non-ionizing   By way of UV rays (240-280 m is bactericidal range)
     Ionising   By way of Gamma rays
     Gases   By way of ethylene oxide
  C. *Chemical:* This is sterilisation of sharp instruments and as an emergency
     Alcohol   By way of ethanol
     Aldehyde   By way of formaldehyde
     Halogen   By way of chlorine
     Phenol   By way of carbolic acid

Q.3 What is Cidex?
Ans. It is glutaraldehyde used for rubber or plastics and to be used for only 15 days from the day of preparation and then it has to made new one.

Q.4 What is dilution of savlon is used?
Ans. It should be 1:1 with water.

Q.5 What agent is used for sterilisation of sutures, needles and blades?
Ans. They should be kept in Lysol for 1-2 hours before use or to be kept in Cidex for same time.

Q.6 How many tablets of formalin are to be used chimko box?
Ans. 4-10 tablets are to be used for 24 hours as they provide formalin vapours.

OT TECHNIQUE AND INFECTIONS

Q.1 What are the causes of contamination in OT?
Ans.
- Entering bacteria by air or direct sedimentation
- Entering many persons in OT and their increased activity
- Maximum concentration is during induction, positioning and extubation

- Due to over use of cautery, and more tissue damage
- General decrease in resistance power by more loss of blood.

Q.2 What are conditions where there is increased risk of infection in OT?

Ans. It is more when there is decreased defence of host such as congenital, old age, obesity, diabetes, rheumatoid arthritis, Implant surgery.

Q.3 What are basic conditions of ideal OT?

Ans.
- People entering OT should wear special and separate pants, suits, shoes with ankle closure, head cover, masks
- UV radiation
- Double gloves security
- Laminar airflow
- Standard and properly sterilised drapes and gowns
- Humidity should be more than 50%
- Air temperature should be 21.1° to 21.4°C
- HEPA filters should be used to clear 99.9% particles
- Proper exhaust.

Q.4 What are sites of bacterial colonisation in polytrauma patients?

Ans. At IV canula sites, at tracheostomy site, at indwelling catheter.

Q.5 What is ASA classification?

Ans. It is risk index score
- Healthy patients
- Mild systemic diseases
- Mild disease with functional impairment
- Severe systemic diseases
- Moribund patients
- 3, 4, 5 are major risk factors in postoperative infection.

SUTURE MATERIALS

Q.1 From where do you get absorbable sutures (non synthetic)?

Ans. They are from cattle, beef cattle and sheep.

Q.2 What is length of time it takes for absorption of gut?

Ans. Tensile strength is lost within 15 days and absorbed in 6–120 days by proteolytic enzymes.

Q.3 What are synthetic absorbable sutures?

Ans. They are:
- Dexon (Green) homopolymer glycolide—90 days
- Vicryl (violet) copolymer glycolide—70 days
- PDS (white)—180 days.

Ward Rounds, Suture Materials, Methods of Sterilisation and OT Techniques 165

Q.4 What is classification of sutures?

Ans. They are two types: (a) Absorbable, and (b) Nonabsorbable, so they are classified as follows:
A. *Monofilament:* Absorbable—surgical gut (plain and chromic catgut) and collagen (plain and chromic)
   Nonabsorbable—polyamide, polypropolene, steel, polyester.
B. *Multifilament:* Absorbable—polyglycolic and polyglactin
   Nonabsorbable—surgical silk, polyester braided, polyamide braided, steel.

Q.5 What are silk, linen and cotton?

Ans.
- *Silk:* Cocoon of silk larvae and protein covered with wax, strength is lost after two years but knots are easy to take.
- *Linen:* Made of flex and cellulose and gains 10% more strength when wet, used as ligatures for pedicles.
- *Cotton:* From seed of cotton but handling is not good and weaker than silk.

Q.6 What are advantages of nylon?

Ans. They are polyamides, minimally reactive, but knot security is low and of good strength can be removed even after 21 days without any problem.

Q.7 What are prolene?

Ans. They are dyed polymer, polyprolene monofilament, has high tensile strength and low tissue reaction.

Q.8 How do you select suture materials and for what?

Ans. They are selected and used for particular areas:
- For skin and tendons, which heal slowly so nonabsorbable sutures are used
- For muscles and peritoneum, absorbable materials are used
- For tissues not to get contamination, avoid multifilament sutures
- For cosmoses, inert material is used
- For closed subcutaneous, polyamides are used
- For cardiovascular surgery, polyprolene and polyester sutures are used
- For pancreatic surgery, nonabsorbable sutures are used
- For microsurgery, 8.0 to 10.0 polyamide monofilament sutures are used
- For orthopaedic surgery, for muscles and fascia absorbable material is used, Polyester steel wire used for THR and tendons
- For postirradiation, polypropylene is used.

Q.9 What are the advantages of eyeless needles?

Ans. They are less traumatic to soft tissues, of uniform strength, sterility is maintained, no accidental unthreading, and for faster and efficient surgery.

Q.10 What are ideal sizes of suture materials for different tissues?

Ans. They are:
- For peritoneum, use absorbable material with sizes of 2.0 to 3.0
- For muscles, use absorbable sizes of 1.0 to 0.1

- For linea alba, silk is better of size 1.0
- For tendons, polyester is being used of size 4.0

Q.11 What are the types of needles used for suturing?
Ans.
- Round body—to avoid damage of tissue, which has tapering end and trocar point
- Cutting needles, used for fascia, skin with conventional and slim blade
- Micropoint needles used for microsurgery.

41
CHAPTER

Miscellaneous Affections

Q.1 What is Dupuytren's contracture?
Ans. It is proliferative fibroplasias of subcutaneous tissue of the palm and fingers leading to progressive flexion contracture.

Q.2 What are fingers, commonly affected?
Ans. Usually, ring and small fingers are affected but sometimes middle finger, thumb or index finger are also involved.

Q.3 Which tissues are affected?
Ans. Mainly fascia of palm and fingers are affected and in addition, there is thinning of subcutaneous fat, thickening and dimpling of overlying skin may occur.

Q.4 What are the other connective tissue disorders associated with Dupuytren's contracture?
Ans. They are: Plantar fibromatosis—Ledderhose's disease
Knuckle pads—Garrod's nodes
Peyronic's disease.

Q.5 What is de Quervain's disease?
Ans. This stenosing tenosynovitis of the first dorsal compartment at the wrist, commonly seen in females between 30 years and 50 years of age.

Q.6 What are the causes of de Quervain's disease?
Ans. This is due to over use of wrist and hand and also seen in cases of inflammatory arthritis. In some patients at first dorsal compartment, there is dividing septum or there is anomalous tendon in third tunnel and these septi may cause stenosis.

Q.7 What is clinical picture of de Quervain's disease?
Ans. Pain and tenderness localised to the radial aspect of wrist and pain becomes worst with movements of thumb as thumb extensor and abductor pass through same compartment.

Q.8 What is treatment of de Quervain's disease?
Ans. Coservative method—rest, immobilisation of thumb and wrist, local steroid injection, systemic anti-inflammatory drugs. If this fails, then surgical release is the choice left.

Q.9 What is intersection syndrome?

Ans. This is tenosynovitis of second dorsal compartment.

Q.10 What is clinical picture of intersection syndrome?

Ans. Pain and swelling 4 cm above the wrist, in severe cases crepitus may be heard, this is due to repetitive use of wrist.

Q.11 What is treatment of intersection syndrome?

Ans. Initial trial of conservative method such as rest, change in work, local steroid injection, which is successful in many cases otherwise surgical release has to be done of second dorsal compartment.

Q.12 What is trigger finger/What is its clinical picture?

Ans. This is stenosing tenosynovitis of flexor tendons of fingers causing catching or triggering of the finger with locking in flexion. They present with pain at proximal interphalangeal joint though the lesion is at metacarpophalangeal joint with or without palpable nodule on the flexor tendon proximal to MCP joint, affecting usually ring and middle fingers usually affecting middle-aged women and neonates, where spontaneous recovery may occur after some age.

Q.13 Where is lesion anatomically?

Ans. The fingers have four annular and three cruciform pulleys, which prevent bowstringing of flexor tendons. When A-1 pulley becomes thickened and narrowed due to chronic inflammation, which entraps the tendon and there is reactive nodular fusiform enlargement of tendon sheath which traps the tendon.

Q.14 What is treatment of trigger finger?

Ans. A trial of splinting and local steroid injection is given, upon failure of this surgical treatment which includes incising:
- A-1 pulley without cutting
- A-2 pulley to avoid bowstringing.

Q.15 What are method of surgical release of trigger finger?

Ans. *Open incision:* A transverse incision is taken on flexor surface of metacarpophalangeal joint and A-1 pulley is cut after identification longitudinally with 15 no. blade.

Percutaneous technique: A 19-gauge needle is advanced one inch to proximal margin of A-1 pulley and cut with tip of needle but there are problems of incomplete cut and tendon damage.

Push knife technique: The knife with straight blade is tapered leading to flanged edge and complete cut is done through 2 mm incision.

Q.16 What is mallet finger? What is its treatment?

Ans. This is flexion deformity of distal interphalangeal joint due to loss of continuity of extensor tendon with distal phalanx or may be due to avulsion of tendon or avulsion fracture at tendon insertion. Treatment by surgery if major portion of fracture fragment is avulsed or splinting is quite enough.

Q.17 What is boxer's fracture? What is treatment?
Ans. It is fracture of neck of fifth metacarpal which is seen commonly in brawlers or persons who strike wall in anger.

Treatment: Minimal immobilisation, closed reduction with pin fixation, open reduction, closed reduction with plaster immobilisation.

Q.18 What is Bennett's fracture? How it is treated?
Ans. This is fracture dislocation of base of first metacarpal joint, described by Edward H Bennett 1882, which includes intra-articular fracture separating volar lip fragment form the metacarpal shaft, which is displaced laterally and dorsally at base of abductor pollicis longus and then pull of this tendon on distal shaft enhances the displacement of the base in abduction.

Treatment: Closed reduction with percutaneous pin fixation of metacarpal to trapezium, open reduction with pin fixation if closed reduction fails, small cortical AO screw can be fixed in place of pin, Joshi's external stabilisation system (JESS) fixator.

Q.19 What is gamekeeper's thumb?
Ans. This is due to injury to ulnar collateral ligament of thumb MCP, which was labelled by Campbell in 1955. This is commonly seen in skiers due to forced abduction of the thumb against planted ski pole, also seen in ball-handling athletes. Actually, skier's thumb is better word to describe this.

Q.20 What are zones of injury of the flexor tendons in the hand and wrist?
Ans. They are:
- *Zone I:* Insertion of FDP at distal phalanx to the middle of middle phalanx,
- *Zone II:* Middle of the middle phalanx to distal palmer crease,
- *Zone III:* Distal palmer crease to distal edge of carpal tunnel,
- *Zone IV:* Carpal tunnel,
- *Zone V:* Proximal edge of the carpal tunnel to the musculocutaneous junction.

Q.21 What is Jersey finger?
Ans. This is avulsion of FDP tendon from its insertion on the distal phalanx, occurring in sportsmen, during forceful flexion causing avulsion. The treatment is of early surgical repair.

Q.22 What is a Boutonniere deformity? How does it occur?
Ans. This progressive condition occurring many times in patients with rheumatoid arthritis where this deformity has three parts: (a) Flexion of PIP joint; (b) Hyperextension of distal interphalangeal (DIP) joint; and (c) Hyperextension of metaphalangeal joint. Due to synovial proliferation within proximal interphalangeal (PIP) joint, stretching of extensor mechanism takes place and

leading to inability to maintain full extension of PIP joint, leading to slipping of lateral tendinous band to volar side which become fixed in same position and there is shortening of oblique retinacular ligament resulting hyperextension and limitation of active flexion. Patients try to compensate for flexion deformity of PIP joint by hyperextending the MP joint. As the deformity is progressive from supply and passively correctable condition to fixed and rigid condition, may be disabling the patient.

Q.23 What is a swan neck deformity?

Ans. This is characterised by hyperextension of PIP joint, flexion of DIP joint and weakening of periarticular structures of PIP joint due to synovitis tightness of intrinsic musculature creates abnormal force across the joint resulting swan neck deformity.

Q.24 What is Kienbock's disease?

Ans. It is due to avascular necrosis of lunate bone resulting in fragmentation and osseous necrosis.

Q.25 What is the cause?

Ans. Exact cause is unknown but it may be due to repeated stress or an acute fracture leading to interruption of blood supply in susceptible or at risk lunate.

Q.26 How do you diagnose Kienbock's disease?

Ans. It is mainly by X-ray, in early stage there is increased density, followed by fracture line, fragmentation and ultimately collapse.
- Stage I—there is linear or compression fracture line of lunate seen by scan or MRI as increased uptake around lunate.
- Stage II—definite increase in density of lunate with some loss of height on radial side at later stage.
- Stage III—there is collapse of lunate in frontal plane but elongation in sagittal plane.
- Stage IV—with all above findings there is generalised carpal degenerative arthritis.

Q.27 What is treatment of Kienbock's disease?

Ans.
- Aim—revascularisation of lunate by different methods
- Stage I—immobilisation is choice, external fixator to prevent compression
- Stage II—equalisation procedure decrease shear and compressive forces, radial or ulnar shortening, give better results
- Stage III—equalisation, limited intercarpal fusion, across midcarpal row
- Stage IV—proximal carpectomy and wrist fusion.

Q.28 What are the common causes of pain in foot?

Ans. Interdigital neuroma, lumbar spine disorders, plantar fasciitis, plantar fibromatosis, peripheral neuritis, tarsal tunnel syndrome, peripheral vascular disease, diabetic neuropathy, tenosynovitis, tarsal coalition, reflex sympathetic dystrophy.

Q.29 What is Morton's Neuroma?
Ans. This is peripheral thickening of the common digital nerve of second or third interspace of foot, usually in females, with unknown etiology but may be due to trauma or extrinsic pressure.

Q.30 What is clinical picture of Morton's neuroma?
Ans. There is presenting symptom is of pain on plantar aspect between metatarsal heads of burning or tingling type, pain in enhanced with wearing of narrow toe box, and pain is relieved by removal of shoe and rest. Manual pressure when applied to forefoot results in click in third web space which is known as Mulder's sign indicating presence of Morton's neuroma.

Q.31 What is treatment of Morton's neuroma?
Ans.
- Conservative treatment—aim to reduce compression of forefoot by wide toe box, firm sole, rigid arch support, metatarsal pads, with anti-inflammatory drugs. With few local injection of local steroids (should not repeat many times).
- Surgical treatment—surgical excision with guarded prognosis.

Q.32 What is tarsal tunnel? What are its contents?
Ans. This is fibro-osseous tunnel formed by flexor retinaculum, medial wall of calcaneum and talus, medial malleolus. The tunnel contains tendons of tibialis posterior, flexor digitorum longus, flexor hallucis and tibial artery, vein and nerve.

Q.33 What is clinical picture of tarsal tunnel syndrome?
Ans. This was first described by Keck in 1962. The aetiology may be due to fracture callus, ganglion of tendon sheaths, lipoma, exostosis, engorged venous plexus, and excessive pronation of hindfoot. Presenting as numbness, diffuse plantar burning, tingling pain increases with activity, relieved with rest, sometimes pain gets radiated along posterior tibial nerve.

The diagnosis is by typical pain, positive Tinel's sign, and positive EMG due to entrapment of posterior tibial nerve or its branches.

Q.34 What is treatment of tarsal tunnel syndrome?
Ans.
- Conservative treatment—non-steroidal anti-inflammatory drugs, local steroid injections, orthotic which limits pronation of hind foot.
- Surgical treatment—release.

Q.35 What is dancer's tendonitis?
Ans. This is stenosing tenosynovitis or tendinitis of flexor hallucis longus (FHL) may be due to direct blunt trauma, previous laceration, repetitive impact, or excessive plantar flexion as in ballet dancer in pointed position.

Q.36 What is clinical picture of flexor-hallucis longus (FHL) tendinitis?

Ans. The stenosing synovitis of FHL occurs at within sheath behind. Medial malleolus, at the start of fibro-osseous tunnel between medial and lateral talar tubercles, or between the hallux sesamoid, presenting pain, swelling, and crepitus posterior to medial malleolus, pain in enhanced by active and passive movements of the hallux interphalangeal joint.

Q.37 What is the treatment of FHL tendonitis?

Ans. Only conservative treatment is sufficient such as NSAIDs, stretching exercises, training modifications, and immobilisation for short-term.

Q.38 What is posterior tibial tendon dysfunction (PTTD)?

Ans. The degenerative changes of the posterior tibial tendon take place at the site of hypovascularity distal to medial malleolus may be due to obesity, diabetes, hypertension, previous trauma, seronegative arthropathies, and steroid exposure.

Q.39 What are stages of PTTD?

Ans.
- Stage I—medial ankle pain and swelling with mild posterior tibial tendon weakness.
- Stage II—disruption of posterior tibial tendon with flexible flat foot deformity.
- Stage III—disruption of posterior tibial tendon with rigid flat foot deformity.

There may be weakness of inversion, and difficulty with single heel raise.

Q.40 What is treatment of PTTD?

Ans.
- Stage I—immobilisation and anti-inflammatory drugs.
- Stage II—orthotics, synovectomy with tendon transfer.
- Stage III—if conservative line fails then fusion of hind foot.

Q.41 What is clinical picture of congenital vertical talus (CVT)?

Ans. This is rigid deformity to be called as convex pes valgus with rigid equines deformity with an everted or valgus heel, marked dorsiflexion, abduction of mid and forefoot creating rocket bottom foot, may be associated with some other congenital deformities such as myelomeningocoele, arthrogryposis multiplex and other syndromes.

Here the extensor tendons and tibialis anterior are contracted, there may be anterior subluxation of peroneal tendons and tibialis posterior, with contracture of dorsal navicular, calcaneocuboid, posterior capsule and calcaneofibular ligament.

Q.42 What is treatment of cerebral venous thrombosis (CVT)?

Ans.
- First—immobilisation in cast.
- Operative release—may be in one stage or two stages. Extensive release has to be done for correction.

Q.43 What is bunion?
Ans. This deformity of great toe presenting as medial prominence and lateral deviation of great toe. Correctly called as hallux valgus.

Q.44 What is hallux valgus?
Ans. This is also lateral deviation of great toe due to lateral subluxation of great toe at MTP joint or may be due to intrinsic deformity within great toe proximal phalanx or at interphalangeal joint. This may be associated with metatarsus primus varus with pronation of great toe.

Q.45 What is aetiology of hallux valgus?
Ans. Heredity, flat feet, metatarsus primus varus, joint hyperlaxity, hypermobile first cuneiform joints, abnormal length of first metatarsal.

Q.46 What is the goal of surgery ? What are the procedures available?
Ans. The primary goal is to improve function and to reduce the pain by restoring normal anatomy of great toe. The available different procedures are:
- Medial eminence resection
- Resection of base of proximal phalanx of great toe—Keller's operation
- Bunionectomy with soft tissue correction at MTP joint
- Bunionectomy with soft tissue procedure and osteotomy of first metatarsal at proximal side—modified McBride operation.
    - Bunionectomy with osteotomy of first metatarsal at distal portion—Chevron operation.
    - Fusion of first metatarsal phalangeal joint
    - Bunionectomy with distal soft tissue procedure and first cuneiform joint arthrodesis—modified Lapidus procedure, 90% people get good result after surgery.

Q.47 What are the complications of operations of metatarsal osteotomy?
Ans.
- Nonunion
- Dorsiflexion at osteotomy
- Plantar flexion at osteotomy
- Shortening of first metatarsal
- Avascular necrosis of metatarsal head.

Q.48 What is osteogenesis imperfecta (OI)?
Ans. It is genetically transmitted disease resulting in fragility of whole skeleton with varying degree of severity, from infant with multiple fractures to child with few fractures before maturity without affecting intelligence.

Q.49 What is aetiology and clinical picture of OI?
Ans. Clinically, the patient has short stature, sclera may be blue in some cases, abnormal thin dentine, multiple deformities of bones, lax ligaments, and impaired hearing.

X-ray shows osteopenia, decrease in mineralisation, thin bony cortices, ill-defined trabeculae, with biconcave vertebrae.

Osteogenesis imperfecta (OI) is due to defect in type I collagen which makes up most of the organic scaffolding for the bone and is also constituent of dentin and sclera and type I collagen plays important role in the components of connective tissue such as ligament and tendons also.

Genetic analysis of collagen from dermal fibroblasts gives side about abnormality of type I collagen. Even DNA testing also helps for diagnosis.

Q.50 What are the types of OI?

Ans. Described by Silence—as follows:
- *Type I:* Mild OI with blue sclera, normal teeth, autosomal dominant.
- *Type II:* Perinatally lethal OI, rarely survive infancy
- *Type III:* Severe progressive deforming OI, dentigenesis imperfecta, neonatal fractures
- *Type IV:* Moderately severe OI sclera fade from blue to white.

Q.51 What is treatment of OI?

Ans. *Medical treatment:* No drug can help but still trials have been made growth hormone which increases height, use of biphosphonate which decrease osteoclastic activity, increase bone density, and bone marrow transplant.

Orthotic support: Braces for lower extremities may help, for spine, ankle and foot, and femur.

Operative treatment: As bone healing is normal in most of the cases, so the fractures have to be treated with immobilisation or internal fixation.
- Sofield operation (1950)—correcting bowing of femur or tibia by multiple osteotomies, realignment of fragments over an intramedullary rod.
- Bailey and Dubow (1963) use of telescopic pair of rods anchoring in each epiphysis of long bone which then expand with growth, indicated in with severely diaphyseal bowing, can be used in upper extremities also.
- Correction by ring fixators with multiple osteotomies (Ilizarov).

Q.52 What is hyperextension deformity of knee?

Ans. Normally, there is 20°–30° flexion deformity of knee upto age of 3 months of newborn babies. But in breech babies, the knees may be hyperextended beyond normal straight position—Genu recouvatum. Where anterior articular surface of tibia have continuous contact with articular surface of distal femur, differentiating from congenital dislocation or subluxation of the knee.

Q.53 What are the types of Genu recurvatum (GR)?

Ans.

A. Physiologic genu recurvatum

B. Pathologic genu recurvatum:
- Grade I—most common (50%), the joint can be passively flexed to 45° to 90°
- Grade II—less common (30%), some articular contact is maintained though tibia is displaced anteriorly, knee flexes upto neutral position with 45° hyperextension.

- Grade III—less common (20%), total displacement of proximal tibia. No articular suface contact, knee is in severe hyperextension with angular deformity of knee.

Q.54 What are the causes and pathology of GR?

Ans. Intrauterine breech presentation is the common cause of genu recurvatum. There may be absence of cruciate ligaments leading to dislocation of knee joint. Some-times, there is fibrosis of quadriceps mechanism. Pathologically, there is lateral subluxation or angular deformity of knee, contraction of the lateral soft tissue structures, hamstrings are displaced anteriorly patellar tendon and quadriceps are contracted, patella is hypoplastic, cruciate ligaments are elongated.

Q.55 What is natural history? What is the treatment of genu racurvatum?

Ans. Usually, genu recurvatum get spontaneously corrected (50%) active treatment is needed for subluxation or dislocation of knee, which may corrected by lengthening of quadriceps and relocation of knee joint.

Initially, gentle active physiotherapy is started. If fails, then closed reduction of subluxation or dislocation is attempted, immobilised by plaster cast for 6–8 weeks, then maintained by orthosis, if this also fails then open surgery is done with lengthening of quadriceps with release of medial and lateral retinaculum, lengthening of patellar tendon insertion, and then immobilised in plaster cast in 90° flexion of knee.

Finally, sometimes there may be restriction of flexion of knee, instability, weak quadriceps, and normal knee after proper treatment.

Q.56 What are the causes of an equines gate?

Ans. They are:
- Congenital—clubfoot
- Idiopathic—gastrocnemius contracture, accessory soleus muscle, generalised triceps contracture
- Neurogenic—cerebral palsy, poliomyelitis
- Myogenic—muscular dystrophy
- Functional—hysterical toe walking.

Q.57 What is flatfoot? What are the types of flatfoot?

Ans. This is foot with depressed medial longitudinal arch. There is sagging of midfoot, valgus alignment of hind foot, abduction of forefoot and over hind foot, supination of fore foot in relation to hind foot.

There are three types of flatfoot:
1. Hypermobile or flexible flatfoot
2. Flexible flatfoot with shortened tendo-Achilles
3. Rigid flatfoot.

Q.58 What are the causes of different types of flatfoot?
Ans.
- *Flexible flatfoot:* Due to laxity of ligaments and shapes of bones of foot, the arch of foot is depressed may be in certain ethnic and racial groups.
- *Rigid flatfoot:* Tarsal coalition, failure of differentiation of and segmentation of primary mesenchyme which form tarsal bones. The most common coalition is between calcaneus and navicular and between talus and calcaneus which may be in the form of fibrous (syndesmosis), cartilaginous (synchodrosis) or osseous (synostosis).

Q.59 What is treatment of different types of flatfoot?
Ans. For flexible flatfoot—surgery is rare, but surgery in done for cases with short tendo-Achilles in the form of lengthening of tendo-Achilles in mild cases, may be associated with osteotomies of corrective deformity or arthrodesis after age of maturity.

For rigid flatfoot—corrective ostotomy for deformity, resection of coalition with interposition of fat, muscle, or tendon is done in children, triple arthrodesis in adults is best choice.

Q.60 What is the cavus foot?
Ans. This is fixed equines deformity of the forefoot in relation to hind foot, leading very high arch of foot, which is usually along medial border of foot, with or without clawing of toes.

Q.61 What are the causes of bilateral cavus foot deformity?
Ans. There are different conditions which are associated with cavus foot:
- Chacot-Marie-Tooth disease
- Polyneuritis
- Spinal muscular dystrophy
- Spinal cord tumor
- Meningomyelocoele
- Syringomyelia
- Muscular dystrophy
- Cerebral palsy
- Idiopathic
- Spinal dysraphism-tethered cord,
- Friedreich's ataxia

Q.62 what is treatment of cavus foot?
Ans. After identifying the deformity, the underlying cause has to searched and to be treated.
- Nonoperative management—has very little role, and this deformity is dynamic and arch support and modification in the shoes may help to some extent.

- Operative management—there are two principles: (a) correction of deformity, and (b) to balance muscle forces.

Correction of deformity—by release of soft tissue, such as release of plantar fascia, abductor hallucis from calcaneum for mild deformity, capsulotomy of talonavicular joint, with release of spring ligament, release of long and short plantar ligament for everted foot, the joints are aligned by soft tissue release, if some deformity is remaining then corrected by osteotomies of medial cuneiform or base of first metatarsal, cuboid or calcaneum, with or without tendon transfer, and arthrodesis in adults with suitable wedge osteotomy.

Q.63 What are the physical findings of bow legs and knock knees?

Ans. *Bow legs:* Normally in standing position with feet together, knees should touch each other. If there is separation and distance between the knees, this condition called bow legs. This may be physiologic also with laxity of ligaments in young children. Progressive asymmetric or unilateral bowing associated with limb length discrepancy should be taken seriously and should be investigated and should be treated.

Knock knees: When the distance between both feet such as intermalleolar distance, is more and knees are closed together, then called knock knees. The gait is of circumduction, there is outward torsion of femur or tibia or both, in severe cases there is lateral tilt and instability of patella. Idiopathic genu valgum may resolve spontaneously. But progressive deformities have to treated with their causes.

Q.64 What are investigations for diagnosis of bow legs and knock knees?

Ans. X-ray: Standing full length X-rays (anteroposterior and lateral) with both knees extended and patellae pointing forward should be taken basically. In dynamic deformities, periodically X-rays should be taken. A plumb line is drawn from the center of femoral head to center of ankle and center of gravity is ascertained. In adolescents, this is mechanical axis which bisects knees and angles made by articular surfaces of the tibia and femur with their respective shafts are also measured.

In patients with symptoms, sunrise view is taken with knees in 30° flexion may reveal patellar tilt of subluxation.

Q.65 What is treatment of both conditions?

Ans. Bow legs—below age of 2 years and knock knees below age of 6 months may resolve spontaneously.

Coservative treatment—use of braces, corrective shoes, exercises, physical therapy, but have no lasting effect.

Operative procedures

Epiphysiodesis: It is aimed to change the angle of the growth and leading to straightening of limb. This can be done either percutaneous or by open method.

Stapling: By placing one or more staples around physis, one can induce an angular change with continued growth and sparing periosteum, the method is reversible means of manipulating growth and it is done for adolescents and in time, the staples are removed.

Osteotomy: Reserved for severe deformities either of femur or tibia and fibula, osteotomy of proximal tibia has advantages of having less complications of compartment syndrome and injury to peroneal nerve. And osteotomies are delayed till skeletal maturity.

Q.66 What is prognosis of these conditions?

Ans. *Bow legs*: If the mechanical axis is medial to knee or in the medial compartment, eccentric and pathologic compression of the medial meniscus and articular cartilage will enhance degenerative process leading to secondary osteoarthritis and in advanced cases, lateral ligament give way to excessive tensile forces and once the articular cartilage has worn away erosion of bone take place.

Knock knees: With significant knock knee deformities, mechanical axis produce pathological compression of lateral compartment combined with tensile stresses on the medial ligaments and shear forces on patella, resulting to patellar tilt and instability leading to degenerative arthritis of patellofemoral joint and lateral compartment of joint.

Q.67 What is Jones fracture?

Ans. This is fracture of proximal fifth metatarsal 1.5 cm from tip of tuberosity, divided into three types such as:
1. Type I—fracture of tuberosity at tarsometatarsal junction
2. Type II—Jones fracture- entering 4–5th intermetatarsal articulation
3. Type III—fracture of proximal diaphysis of 5th metatarsal.

Q.68 What are the compartments of foot?

Ans. There are nine separate compartments of the foot:
- Medial compartment contains adductor hallucis and flexor hallucis brevis muscles.
- Lateral compartment having abductor digiti minimi and flexor digiti minimi brevis muscles
- Deep central compartment having quadratus plantar muscle
- Superficial central compartment having flexor digitorum brevis muscle a separate fascial compartment in each intermetatarsal space having plantar interosseous muscles
- Distal medial plantar forefoot having oblique head of abductor hallucis muscle.

Q.69 What is classification of ankle sprains?

Ans.
- *Grade I:* Negative anterior drawer and talar tilt test
- *Grade II:* Positive anterior/negative talar tilt test
- *Grade III:* Positive anterior drawer and talar tilt test.

Q.70 What is talar tilt test?

Ans. Performed by grasping the foot and ankle during inverting the talus over tibia. This is for integrity of calcaneofibular ligament and anterior talofibular ligament. Normally, it is less than 5° and with stress X-rays give some clue.

Q.71 What is treatment for ankle sprains?

Ans. Grade I—rest, ice compression, and elevation with protected weight bearing, and early mobilization and sometimes bracing may be needed.

Grade II—protected weight bearing, isometric or kinetic exercises, and supportive braces for 6 months at least during sports. Proprioceptive rehabilitation includes joint positioning, activities, to convert conscious programming to unconscious to get awareness of joint sense and to regain reflex to prevent injury again stability.

Q.72 What is treatment for acute compartment syndrome?

Ans. Emergency release of all four compartments of leg such as anterior, lateral, superficial posterior and deep posterior should be done through lateral or medial or both incisions.

Q.73 What are methods of treatment of fracture of tibia?

Ans. *Simple fractures:*

Conservative method: Closed reduction and plaster casting in low energy fractures, from groin to foot and for 6-8 weeks, or till fracture heals, after acceptable reduction such as less than 1 cm shortening, less than 50 angulation in any plane, less than 100 malrotation, and more than 50% cortical apposition, or walking plaster (Sermionto).

Operative treatment: Indicated in failure of closed reduction, multiple trauma, ipsilateral femoral fracture, bilateral tibial fractures, fractures with compartment syndrome, fractures with vascular injuries, and pathologic fractures and for early rehabilitation, They are in the form of plating, (simple or compression), intramedullary nailing such as V nailing. Ender's nailing, K nailing, interlocking nailing either static or dynamic such as AO nailing (static) or Daga interlocking nailing (dynamic), Grosse-Kemf nailing, Frankfurt nailing, the nailing may be reamed or unreamed.

Compound fractures: Either primary nailing or external fixators in the form of ring fixators-Ilizarov or tubular fixators.

Q.74 How do you treat infection of tibia?

Ans. By irrigation and debridement of all necrotic tissues, removal of hardware of fracture has healed, or if implant is loose, in that case, change of implant is indicated, for healing of fracture and with proper antibiotics, and osteotomy of fibula, if that is healed and tibial fracture has not healed.

Q.75 What is true and apparent leg length discrepancy?

Ans. *True leg length discrepancy:* Measurable difference of lengths of two lower limbs from anterior superior iliac spine (ASIS) to medial malleolus with keeping both lower limbs in same anatomical attitude.

Apparent leg length discrepancy: This is measurable difference in two lower limbs from umbilicus or xiphisternum to the medial malleolus.

Q.76 What is functional leg length discrepancy?

Ans. This is assessed by putting blocks under short leg so as to level pelvis while standing. This, most important from the point of further treatment.

Q.77 How leg length discrepancy (LLD) is assessed?

Ans. *Clinically:* (a) by leveling pelvis and blocks under short leg; (b) measuring the distance from ASIS to medial malleolus; (3) distance is measured from umbilicus or xiphisternum to medial malleolus; and (4) Galeazzi's sign.

Radilologically: (a) By Scanogram, (b) Teleroentgenogram, (c) CT scan, (4) Orthoroentgenogram.

Q.78 What is Galeazzi's sign?

Ans. The patient is in supine position with flexion of knees and feet, and if the knees are at different level. Then one limb is shorter.

Q.79 What is scanogram?

Ans. The series of X-rays are taken of hips, knees, ankles with radiographical measuring tape to avoid magnification and the lengths are measured but with contracture of hips and knees can give false impression.

If the scanogram is taken with lateral or posteroanterior position of leg, then errors of contractures of hips and knees can be rectified.

Q.80 What is an orthoroentgenogram?

Ans. This is 3-feet X-ray taken in three separate exposures with beam over joints to avoid magnification error.

Q.81 What is a teleroentgenogram?

Ans. This is single 3 feet X-ray taken of lower extremity giving idea about malalignment or lesions of bone in X-ray and measurement is not distorted by movements of patient with disadvantage of difficulty in storage of such large film.

Q.82 What are the causes of acquired LLD?

Ans. Congenital—hemihypertrophy, congenital short femur, fibular hemimelia, hips dislocation, proximal femoral focal deficiency, posteromedial bowing of legs.

Acquired—Traumatic—femoral or tibial length malunion, or over growth, growth due to fracture of plate.

Paralytic—Polio, cerebral palsy.

Vascular—hemangioma, Klippel-Trenaunay-Weber syndrome.

Neoplastic—Wilm's tumor, radiation treatment, infectious.

Q.83 Why there is over growth after fracture?
Ans. There may be local hyperemia induced by fracture healing and remodeling.

Q.84 What are problems of LLD?
Ans. Negligible LLD does not cause any problem (less than 1 cm) but more than 1 cm LLD can cause:
- Inefficient gait—if the LLD is larger than gait becomes less efficient
- Cosmetic problem—apparent look is good
- Arthritis—as longer leg is less covered may be predisposed to early arthritic changes
- Backache, functional scoliosis.

Q.85 What are guidelines for selection of patients for treatment?
Ans. LLD at maturity:

Less than 2 cm	No treatment is needed
2–6 cm	Raise in shoes, epiphyseodesis, or shortening of femur to equalize leg lengths
6–20 cm	Lengthening limb, or combination of lengthening and shortening with or without any additional procedure such as stapling or epiphyseodesis
More than 20 cm	Amputation and prosthetic fitting.

Q.86 What is contribution of femur and tibia for growth?
Ans.
- Femur—Proximal femur-30% and distal femur—70%
- Tibia—Proximal-55% and distal tibia—45%.

Q.87 What are the operations available for leg lengthening?
Ans. Simple devices—half pin external fixators attached to large threaded pins, such as Wagner and orthofix devices.

Complex devices—base on distraction principle, allow rotation or angular changes, they are attached to bone by thin tension wires, inserted through limb and these wires are attached to rings, even by slowly and gradually complex deformities can be corrected and bone is lengthened such as Ilizarov, Russian scientist and Monticelli-Spinelli devices.

The lengthening should be at rate of 1 mm per day to avoid over stretching of nerves and vessels and give them chance for better regeneration.

The external fixators should be used for 60 days for lengthening and 120 days for bone maturity in addition. During limb lengthening, hypertension may occur so monitoring of blood pressure of patient should be done periodically. And during hypertension phase lengthening should be stopped till blood pressure comes to normal and again lengthening should be started.

Q.88 What are advantages of limb lengthening?
Ans. Two clear advantages are seen:
1. Operation is done on shorter limb which is accepted by parents and patient.
2. Finally good height is achieved to equalise the lengths.

Q.89 What are complications of limb lengthening?
Ans. They are:
- Incomplete cardiectomy or osteotomy
- Irritation and infection at insertion of pins
- Cotractures ankle or knee or dislocations of joint—hip or knee
- Premature consolidation
- There may be new deformity due to regeneration of bone
- Hypertension
- Breakage of pins or cut out
- Failure to get desired length
- Osteomyelitis
- Fracture or deformity in the regenerate following removal of device
- Premature spontaneous closure or accelerated physical growth.

Q.90 What are the pitfalls in the treatment of LLD?
Ans.
- Arithmetic mistake so proper and correct calculations should be done
- Correcting current discrepancy in growing child instead of the predicted discrepancy at maturity
- Short pelvis or hind foot due to polio should be taken into account
- Proper calculation and anticipation of growth should be done. If not then proper result will not be there.

42 CHAPTER

Commonly Accepted Classifications in Orthopaedics

Q.1 What is Boyd's classification of congenital pseudoarthrosis of tibia?
Ans.
- *Type I:* Anterior bowing and congenital pseudoarthrosis
- *Type II:* Anterior bowing with hour glass constriction
- *Type III:* Bone cyst with or without fracture
- *Type IV:* Sclerosis with or without bone loss
- *Type V:* Associated with defect in fibula
- *Type VI:* Interosseous neurofibroma.

Q.2 What is Orthopaedic Trauma Association (OTA) classifications of fractures?
Ans.
- *Linear:*
  - Transverse
  - Oblique
  - Spiral
- *Comminuted:*
  - Less than 50%
  - Greater than 50%
  - With butterfly fragment less than 50%
  - Butterfly fragment more than 50%
- *Segmental:*
  - Two levels
  - Three or more level
  - Longitudinal split
  - Comminuted
- *Bone loss:*
  - Less than 50%
  - More than 50%
  - Complete bone loss.

Q.3 What is Gustillo's classifications of compound fractures?
Ans. It classified as:
- Open fracture with clean wound less than 1 cm.
- Laceration more than 1 cm long without extensive soft tissue damage, skin flaps or avulsions.

- Open fracture with extensive soft tissue damage but with adequate soft tissue coverage of bone having segmental or severe comminution.
- Open fracture with extensive soft tissue loss with periosteal stripping where bone is exposed.
- Open fracture with vascular injuries which need repair.

Q.4 How patellar fractures are classified?
Ans. They are undisplaced and displaced (a) transverse, (b) vertical, (c) oblique.

Q.5 What is Dannis-Weber AO classification of ankle fractures?
Ans. This is based on fracture of fibula:

Type A: Fracture of fibula below the level of syndesmosis
- Isolated fracture
- With fracture of medial malleolus
- With fracture of posterior malleolus

Type B: Fracture of fibula at the level of syndesmosis
- Isolated
- With injury to deltoid ligament or to medial malleolus
- With associated medial lesion and fracture of posterior lateral tibia

Type C: Fracture of fibula above the level of syndesmosis
- Isolated fibular fracture
- Comminuted fibular fracture
- Proximal fibular fracture.

Q.6 What is Lauge Hansen's classification of ankle fractures?
Ans. This classification is based upon the suspected mechanism of injury. In every category, the injury begins with specific anatomical location and progresses around ankle in sequence the patterns are created.

Supination adduction:
- Transverse avulsion fracture of fibula below the level of tibial plafond
- Vertical fracture of medial malleolus.

Supination external rotation:
- Rupture of anterior tibiofibular ligament
- Spiral fracture of distal fibula
- Fracture of posterior malleolus or rupture of posterior tibiofibular ligament
- Oblique fracture of medial malleolus or rupture of deltoid ligament.

Pronation adduction:
- Transverse fracture of medial malleolus
- Rupture of syndesmosis ligament
- Short oblique or horizontal fracture of fibula above the level of ankle joint.

Pronation external rotation:
- Transverse fracture of medial malleolus or rupture of deltoid ligament
- Disruption of anterior tibiofibular ligament
- Oblique fracture of fibula, 4–5 cm above level of tibial plafond

- Rupture of posterior tibiofibular ligament or avulsion fracture of posterior lateral tibia.

Pronation dorsiflexion (PD)
- Fracture of medial malleolus
- Fracture of anterior tibial margin
- Supramalleolar fracture of tibia
- Transverse fracture of posterior tibial surface.

Q.7 How fractures of talus are classified?

Ans. Here Hawkins classification system is used:
- *Type I:* Undisplaced vertical fracture of talus
- *Type II:* Displaced fracture of talar neck with subluxation or dislocation of subtalar joint with intact ankle joint
- *Type III:* Displaced fracture of talar neck with dislocation of the body of talus from subtalar and ankle joints
- *Type IV:* Very rare-dislocation of talar head where there is great risk of AVN.

Q.8 What is Brenda and Harry's classification of osteochondral fracture of talus?

Ans.
- *Stage I:* Small area of subchondral compression
- *Stage II:* Partially detached ligament
- *Stage III:* Completely detached fragment remaining in crater
- *Stage IV:* Detached fragment lying loose in the joint.

Q.9 What is Holland More classification of fracture dislocation of upper end of tibia?

Ans. This is as follows:
- Type I—coronal split fracture
- Type II—entire condylar fracture
- Type III—rim avulsion fracture
- Type IV—rim compression fracture
- Type V—four part fracture.

Q.10 How Muller has classified fracture of distal end of femur?

Ans. This is as follows:

Type A   *Fracture involving distal shaft of femur*
Type B   *Condylar fractures:*
    B1 Sagittal split of lateral condyle
    B2 Sagittal split of medial condyle
    B3 Fracture in coronal plane
Type C   *T and Y condylar fractures:*
    C1 Uncomminuted
    C2 Comminuted fracture shaft with two principal articular fragments
    C3 Fracture having intra-articular comminution.

Q.11 What is Tronzo's classification of inter-trochanteric fracture neck of femur?
Ans.
- *Type I:* Undisplaced and incomplete fracture
- *Type II:* Undisplaced and complete fracture
- *Type III:* Displaced proximal fragment breaking into distal fragment medullary cavity with exploded posterior wall
- *Type IV:* Displaced and proximal fragment shifted medially
- *Type V:* Reversal intertrochanteric fracture.

Q.12 What is Boyd and Griffin classification of intertrochanteric fracture?
Ans.
- Type I—fracture extending along intertrochanteric line from greater trochanter to lesser trochanter
- Type II—comminuted fracture beginning along intertrochanteric line
- Type III—subtrochanteric fracture with fracture of lesser trochanter
- Type IV—fracture of trochanteric region with proximal shaft in two planes.

Q.13 What is Evans classification of IT fracture?
Ans. Type I Undisplaced (stable)
         Displaced but reduced
         Displaced but not reduced
         Comminuted
     Type II Reversed obliquity (unstable).

Q.14 What is OTA (Orthopaedic Trauma Association) alphanumeric fracture classification of IT Fracture?
Ans.

31-A	Femur-proximal trochanteric
31-A1	Pertrochanteric simple
31-A1.1	Along intertrochanteric line
31-A1.2	Through greater trochanter
31-A1.3	Below lesser trochanter
31-A2	Pertrochanteric multifragmentary
31-A2.1	With one intermediate fragment
31-A2-2	With several intermediate fragments
31-A2.3	Extending more than 1 cm below lesser trochanter
31-A2.3	Intertrochanteric
31-A3.1	Simple oblique
31-A3.2	Simple transverse
31-A3.3	Multifragmentary.

Q.15 What is AO classification of intertrochanteric fracture of femur?
Ans.
A-1 Fracture along with trochanteric line
A-2 Multifragmentary pertrochanteric fracture
A-3 Simple transverse intertrochanteric fracture.

Commonly Accepted Classifications in Orthopaedics   **187**

Q.16 What is Garden's classification of fracture neck of femur?
Ans.
- *Stage I:* Incomplete or impacted fracture neck of femur
- *Stage II:* Complete fracture neck of femur without displacement
- *Stage III:* Complete fracture with partial displacement
- *Stage IV:* Fracture with complete displacement.

Q.17 What is AO classification of fracture neck of femur?
Ans.
- B.1—subcapital fracture with little displacement
- B.2—transcervical fracture neck of femur
- B.3—non impacted displaced subcapital fracture.

Q.18 What is Pauwell's classification of fracture neck of femur?
Ans.
- *Type I:* Pauwells angle less than 30°
- *Type II:* Angle is between 30–50°
- *Type III:* Angle is between 50–70°

Q.19 What is Fielding's classification of subtrochanter is fracture?
Ans.
- *Type I:* At the level of lesser trochanter
- *Type II:* Fracture at between 2.5 and 5 cm below lesser trochanter
- *Type III:* Fracture at between 5 and 7.5 cm below lesser trochanter.

Q.20 What is Seinsheimer's classification of subtrochanteric fracture?
Ans.
- *Type I:* Undisplaced fracture
- *Type II:* Two parts fracture
- *Type III:* Three parts fracture
- *Type IV:* Comminuted fracture with 3 or more fragments
- *Type V:* Subtrochanteric intertrochanteric configuration.

Q.21 What is Thomson and Epstein classification of posterior dislocation of hip?
Ans.
- *Type I:* With or without minor fracture
- *Type II:* With large single fracture of posterior acetabular rim
- *Type III:* Comminution of posterior acetabular rim with or without major fragment
- *Type IV:* Associated with fracture of acetabular roof
- *Type V:* With fracture of femoral head

Q.22 What is Pepkin's classification of type V Thomson Epstein classification?
Ans.
- *Type I:* Posterior dislocation with fracture of head caudal to fovea centralise
- *Type II:* Posterior dislocation with fracture head cephalad to fovea centralise

- *Type III:* Posterior. Dislocation with fracture of head with fracture of neck of femur
- *Type IV:* Posterior dislocation with fracture head with fracture of acetabulum

Q.23 What is Colona's classification of hip fractures in children?

Ans. *Type I:* Trans-epiphyseal separation with or without displacement
Type II: Trancervical fracture with or without displacement
Type III: Basicervical fracture with or without displacement
Type IV: Inter trochanteric fracture

Q.24 What is Ratliff's classification of avascular necrosis of head of femur in children?

Ans.
- *Type I:* Involvement of total head
- *Type II:* Segmental involvement
- *Type III:* Involvement from fracture line to epiphyseal plate.

Q.25 What is Winquist Hansen's classification of comminution of fractures?

Ans.
- *Type I:* Comminuted small piece of bone which is broken
- *Type II:* More than 50% cortical contact
- *Type III:* Less than 50% cortical contact
- *Type IV:* Has no fixed contact with minor proximal and distal fragments
- *Type V:* Segmental transverse fracture
- *Type VI:* Segmental oblique and comminuted fracture
- Type *VII:* Spiral fracture
- *Type VIII:* Proximal transverse fracture
- *Type IX:* Proximal oblique fracture
- *Type X:* Proximal comminuted fracture
- *Type XI:* Distal transverse fracture
- *Type XII:* Distal oblique fracture
- *Type XIII:* Distal comminuted fracture.

Q.26 how do you classify fracture of olecranon?

Ans.
- *Type I:* Fracture involving proximal 1/3rd of articular surface
- *Type II:* Fracture of middle third of olecranon
- *Type III:* Fracture of distal third of olecranon.

Q.27 What is Mason's classification of fracture of radial head?

Ans.
- *Type I:* Segmental fracture without displacement
- *Type II:* Segmental fracture with displacement
- *Type III:* Comminuted fracture
- *Type IV:* Fracture similar to type III with dislocation of elbow.

Q.28 What is Bado's classification of Monteggia fracture dislocation?
Ans.
- Type I—fracture of middle or proximal third of ulna with anterior dislocation of radial, head with anterior angulation of ulna
- Type II—fracture of middle third or proximal third of ulna with posterior dislocation of radial head with fracture of it
- Type III—fracture of ulna distal to coronoid process with lateral dislocation of radial head
- Type IV—fracture of proximal or middle third of ulna, anterior dislocation of radial head and fracture of proximal third of radius below bicipital groove.

Q.29 What is Salter-Harris classification of epiphyseal injuries?
Ans.
- *Type I:* Epiphyseal separation through epiphyseal plate with or without displacement
- *Type II:* Fractures have metaphyseal spike attached to separated epiphysis with separation through epiphyseal plate
- *Type III:* Separation of epiphyseal plate with fracture through epiphysis into the joint
- *Type IV:* Fracture are through metaphysis, epiphyseal plate, epiphysis into the joint
- *Type V:* Compression fracture of epiphyseal plate where permanent damage is done to plate
- *Type VI:* Bruise or contusion to the periphery of epiphyseal plate.

Q.30 What is Wilkin's classification of fracture of neck of radius in children?
Ans.
- Salter-Harris type II fracture
- Salter-Harris type IV fracture
- Salter-Harris type I fracture.

Q.31 What is Badelon's classification for fracture of lateral condyle of humerus in children?
Ans.
- Type I—Undisplaced fracture
- Type II—Fracture with minimal displacement
- Type III—Fracture with displacement more than 2 mm
- Type IV—Severely displaced with complete separation of fracture edges.

Q.32 What is Milch classification of fracture of lateral condyle of humerus?
Ans.
- Type I—fracture line passes laterally to the trochlea through and into the capitellar- trochlea groove
- Type II—fracture line extends into area of trochlea and produces instability not displaced, moderately displaced and completely displaced.

Q.33 What is classification of fracture of capitellum?
Ans.
- Type I—small shell of bone and articular cartilage
- Type II—large fragment of bone and articular cartilage
- Type III—comminuted fracture.

Q.34 What is Kilfoyle's classification of medial condyle of humerus in children?
Ans.
- Type I—impacted
- Type II—intra-articular and epiphyseal fracture
- Type III—entire medial condyle is displaced.

Q.35 What is Neer's classification of proximal humerus (Humeral head)?
Ans.
- Fracture of anatomical neck of humerus
- Fracture of surgical neck of humerus
- Fracture of greater tuberosity of humerus
- Fracture of lesser tuberosity of humerus
- Fracture dislocation.

Q.36 What is three part fracture?
Ans. Fracture of surgical neck with greater tuberosity with dislocation.

Q.37 What is Riseborough and Radins classification of intercondylar fracture of lower third of humerus?
Ans.
- *Type I:* Undisplaced fracture extending between capitellum and trochlea
- *Type II:* Displaced T or Y fracture, extending from the groove on articular surface of trochlea proximally condyles then dividing transversely or obliquely across the shaft and separating from each other and shaft
- *Type III:* Fracture with rotational displacement of the condyle
- *Type IV:* Fracture with severe comminution of the articular surface and wide separation of condyles.

Q.38 How do you classify the supracondylar fracture of humerus in children by method of Gartland?
Ans.
- *Type I:* Fracture without displacement.
- *Type II:* Fracture with displacement with intact posterior cortex.

Q.39 What is Rockwood's classification of acromioclavicular injuries in children?
Ans.
- *Type I:* Contusion of joint
- *Type II:* Injury to acromioclavicular ligament only

Commonly Accepted Classifications in Orthopaedics **191**

- *Type III:* Rupture of acromioclavicular ligament with intact coracoclavicular ligament
- *Type IV:* Similar to type III with displacement of clavicle posteriorly.
- *Type V:* Disruption of acromioclavicular ligament, coracoclavicular ligament but attached to periosteal sleeve with unstable clavicle, lateral end buried in trapezius muscle.

Q.40 What is classification of Meyr's and Mckeever of intercondylar fracture of tibial eminence?

Ans.
- Type I—undisplaced avulsion fracture.
- Type II—fracture elevated anteriorly and proximally with some displacement with cartilaginous hinge.

Q.41 What is Watson Jones classification of fracture of tibial tuberosity in older children?

Ans.
- *Type I:* Small piece of fracture displaced superiorly
- *Type II:* Fracture at the junction of primary and secondary ossification centers
- *Type III:* Fracture involving epiphyseal plate and proximal articular surface of tibia.

Q.42 What are types of nonunions of fractures?

Ans.
- *Hypertrophic:*
  - Elephant foot nonunion
  - Horse hoof type nonunion
  - Oligotrophic nonunion
- *Atrophic:*
  - Torsion wedge type nonunion
  - Comminuted type nonunion
  - Defect type nonunion
  - Atrophic type nonunion.

Q.43 What is Paley's classification of nonunion of fractures (Ilizarov)?

Ans.

Type A: Bone loss less than 1 cm
    A-1   Mobile
    A-2   Non-mobile
    A-3   No deformity
    A-4   Fixed deformity
Type B: Bone loss more than 1 cm
    B-1   Bony defect and no shortening
    B-2   No bony defect and shortening
    B-3   Bony defect with shortening.

Q.44 How gradation of chodromalacia of patella is done?
Ans.
- Grade I—minimal articular changes with local softening and break in the surface
- Grade II—area of fissuring and irregular surface
- Grade III—definite fissuring extended to subchondral bone
- Grade IV—disappearance of articular cartilage, with exposure and erosion of subchondral bone.

Q.45 What is Watanabe classification of discoid meniscus?
Ans. *Complete type*—entire articular surface of tibial condyle is covered by thickened abnormal meniscus.
Incomplete type—entire articular surface of condyle is not covered and intermediate segment between anterior and posterior horns may vary in thickness and area of coverage of articular surface.
Wrisberg ligament type—it is large cartilaginous posterior horn which has no definite attachment to tibial plateau and entire posterior portion of meniscus is hypermobile.

Q.46 What is Lisfranc's joint?
Ans. Tarsal metatarsal joint is called Lisfranc's joint.

Q.47 What are injuries to Lisfranc's joint?
Ans. They are:
Type A   Total incongruity
Type B   Partial incongruity
             1. medial dislocation
             2. lateral dislocation
Type C   Divergent
             Total displacement
             Partial displacement

Q.48 How do you classify tibial hemimelia?
Ans. There four types of tibial hemimelia—Lloyd Roberts classification:
- Type I—no tibia—some patients may develop upper tibia in the first year of life (delayed ossification)
- Type II—has upper tibia
- Type III—has lower tibia
- Type IV—congenital diastasis of the ankle.

The incidence is one in million

Q.49 How proximal femoral focal deficiency is classified?
Ans. Paley's classification is most recent one which is accepted
- *Type I:* Intact femur with mobile hip and knee with delayed ossification leading to short femur may be absence of femoral neck

- *Type II:* Mobile pseudoarthrosis (a) mobile femoral head and mobile knee (b) stiff or absent femoral head and mobile knee.
- *Type III:* Diaphyseal deficiency of femur (a) partially mobile knee more than 45° (b) stiff knee less than 45°
- *Type IV:* Acetabulum, femoral head, proximal femur are totally absent.

Q.50 What is Heckle's classification of radial dysplasia?
Ans.
- *Type I:* Short distal radius
- *Type II:* Hypoplastic radius
- *Type III:* Partial absence of radius
- *Type IV:* Total absence of radius.

Q.51 What is Swanson's classification of ulnar deficiencies?
Ans.
- *Type I:* Hypoplasia or partial absence of ulna
- *Type II:* Total defect of ulna
- *Type III:* Partial defect of ulna with humeroradial sync
- *Type IV:* Total or partial defect of ulna with congenital amputation of wrist.

Q.52 What is Flatt's classification of cleft hand (central deficiencies)?
Ans.
- *Group O:* All bones are present
- *Group I:* One ray is affected
- *Group II:* Two rays are affected
- *Group III:* Three rays are affected.

Q.53 What is Wassel's classification of thumb polydacyly?
Ans.
- *Type I:* Bifid distal phalanx
- *Type II:* Duplicated distal phalanx
- *Type III:* Bifid proximal phalanx
- *Type IV:* Duplicated proximal phalanx
- *Type V:* Bifid metacarpal
- *Type VI:* Duplicated metacarpal
- *Type VII:* Triphalangism.

Q.54 What is classification of fracture of shaft of femur with femoral head prosthesis?
Ans.
- Type I—spiral fracture which begins proximal to tip of prosthesis and position of fragments are maintained at distal end
- Type II—fracture at the level of tip of stem of prosthesis
- Type III—fracture below the tip of stem of prosthesis.

Q.55 What is Tile and Pennal mechanical classification of pelvic fractures?
Ans.
- Type I—the anteroposterior compression (open book), this is not grossly unstable, where injury hinges the pelvis open on intact posterosuperior SI ligaments.
- Type II—the lateral compression injury occurs due to direct force to iliac crests. Stability depends upon magnitude of force and degree of disruption of posterior pelvic arch.
- Type III—vertical shear injury- where the forces are directed through femur to pelvic ring causing disruption of SI joint. If the displacement is of 1 cm or 0.5 cm vertically of hemipelvis indicating instability.

Q.56 What is Key and Conwell classification of fractures of pelvis?
Ans.
- *Type I—fracture without break in continuity of pelvic ring:*
   a. Avulsion fracture
      1. Anterior superior iliac spine
      2. Anterior inferior iliac spine
      3. Ishial tuberosity
   b. Fracture of pubis or ishium
   c. Fracture of wing of ilium
   d. Fracture of sacrum or coccyx
- *Type II—single break in pelvic ring:*
   a. Fracture of two ipsilateral rammi
   b. Fracture of near or subluxation of symphysis of pubis
   c. Fracture of near or subluxation of SI joint
- *Type III—double break in pelvic ring:*
   a. Double vertical fracture or dislocation of pelvis
   b. Double vertical fracture or dislocation
   c. Severe multiple fractures
- *Type IV—fracture of acetabulum:*
   a. Small fragment associated with dislocation of hip
   b. Linear fracture associated with undisplaced pelvic fracture
   c. Linear fracture with hip joint instability
   d. Fracture secondary to central dislocation of hip.

Q.57 What is Malgaigne fracture?
Ans. Malgaigne fractures are referred as unstable fracture dislocation of pelvis. This fracture includes fractures of all pubic bones such as both superior and inferior rami or dislocation of pubic symphysis, sacral fracture, iliac fracture or dislocation of SI joint. There may be limb length discrepancy, migration of hip, the treatment is open reduction with internal fixation or stabilization with external fixator with open reduction is now-a-days choice of treatment.

Q.58 How fractures of acetabulum are classified?

Ans. The Letournel classification includes ten types of fracture

Type I to V—elementary simple fracture, part or all of one column of acetabulum has been detached elementary fractures include: (1) Posterior column fracture; (2) anterior column fracture; (3) anterior wall fracture; (4) posterior wall fracture; and (5) transverse fracture.

Type VI to X are complex fractures with elementary fractures such as: (1) fracture of the posterior column and posterior wall; (2) associated transverse fracture and posterior wall fracture; (3) T-shaped fracture; (4) associated anterior and posterior hemitransverse fractures and (5) fractures of both columns

Q.59 What is Odgen's classification for acute dislocation of superior tibiofibular joint?

Ans.
- *Type I:* Subluxation
- *Type II:* Anterolateral dislocation
- *Type III:* Posterolateral dislocation
- *Type IV:* Superior dislocation.

Q.60 What is Frykman's classification of fractures of lower end of radius and ulna?

Ans.
- *Type I:* Extra articular fracture of radius only
- *Type II:* Extra articular fracture of radius and ulna
- *Type III:* Fracture of radius extending into radiocarpal joint
- *Type IV:* Fracture of radius and ulna extending into radiocarpal joint
- *Type V:* Fracture of radius involving radioulnar joint
- *Type VI:* Fracture of radius and ulna involving radioulnar joint
- *Type VII:* Fracture of radius involving both joints
- *Type VIII:* Fracture of radius and ulna involving both joints.

Q.61 What is Tsuge classification of Volkman's ischemic contracture?

Ans.
- Mild contracture—wrist flexors contracted but not paralysed
- Moderate contracture—long flexors and wrist flexors are affected
- Severe contracture—flexors and extensors are affected with forearm and fracture of forearm bones with scars of skin with sensory disturbances.

Q.62 What is D'Ambrosia classification of cervical trauma?

Ans.
I—soft tissue injury or disc injury or both
- Without neurological deficit
- With neurological deficit
    - Root signs
    - Cord signs

II—Bony fracture or dislocation without neurological deficit
- Stable
- Unstable

III—Bony fracture or dislocation with neurological deficit
- Complete cord lesion
- *Incomplete cord lesion:*
  - Anterior cord syndrome
  - Central cord syndrome
  - Brown Squared syndrome
  - Nerve root injury.

Q.63 What is Sunder land classification of nerve injury?

Ans.
- I Degree—conduction along axon is interrupted at site of injury physiologically with intact axons with affection of motor function.
- II Degree—disruption of axons with wallerian degeneration distal to site of injury with intact endoneural tube with schwan cells with loss of motor, sensory and sympathetic function.
- III Degree—axon with schwann cell sheath, with disruption of endoneural tube with intact perineurium with neurological deficit.
- IV Degree—funiculi and endoneurium are disrupted, some of epineurium and perineurium preserved but prognosis is poor for return of function.
- V Degree—loss of continuity of nerve trunk in cases of compound fractures with permanent damage without any possibility of recovery.

Q.64 What is Singh and Maini's classification of osteoporosis?

Ans.
- *Grade 6*—well mineralised bone with distinct visible all trabeculae
- *Grade 5*—minimal osteoporosis, secondary to decreased trabeculae which are discontinued
- *Grade 4*—loss of trochanteric trabeculae
- *Grade 3*—primary tension trabeculae are decreased in number and discontinued
- *Grade 2*—decrease in primary tensile and compression trabeculae.

Q.65 What is Catterall's classification of Perthe's disease?

Ans.
- Group I—with no metaphyseal reaction, sequestrum and subchongral fracture line.
- Group II—metaphyseal reaction over antero lateral aspect of head, sequestrum present, and with presence of fracture line over anterior half of head of femur.
- Group III—large sequestrum seen, sclerotic metaphyseal reaction which is diffused on anterolateral area and fracture line is present over posterior half of head of femur.
- Group IV—involvement of whole head, central or diffused metaphyseal reaction with remodeling posterior head of femur.

Q.66 What is Essex-Lopresti classification of fractures of calcaneum?
Ans.
- Type I—by vertical compression force lateral process of talus is driven inferiorly into calcaneum.
- Type II—tongue shaped fracture, with secondary fracture line passes into posterior border of tuberosity where superior surface of body of calcaneum and lateral half of articular surface in included.
- Type III—displaced anterior end dips into cancellous bone of body and posterior end overrides superiorly where primary fracture line opens up inferiorly.
- Type IV—secondary fracture line runs posterior to the joint and there is joint depression.
- Type V—joint fragment is displaced into cancellous body of calcaneum inside the lateral cortex
- Type VI—tuberosity is driven superiorly with loss of tuber angle and primary fracture line is spread over.

Q.67 What is Warwick and Bremmer classification of fracture of Calcaneum?
Ans.
- *Type I—fracture of calcaneum not involving subtalar joint:*
  - Vertical fracture of tuberosity
  - Horizontal fracture of tuberosity
  - Fracture of sustentaculum tali
  - Fracture of anterior end of calcaneum
- *Type II—fracture involving subtalar joint:*
  - Fracture adjacent to subtalar joint without entering into it
  - Fracture with displacement of lateral part of subtalar joint
  - Fracture with involvement of central part of subtalar joint
  - Fracture with crushing over subtalar joint with calcaneocuboid joint.

Q.68 What is McLaughlin's classification of complete rupture of shoulder cuff?
Ans.
- Pure transverse rupture
- Pure longitudinal tear
- Tears with retraction
- Massive avulsion of the cuff.

Q.69 How bony tumours are classified?
Ans.
Type I— tumors of osseous origin:
- Cartilagenous—osteochondroma
  Chondroma
  Chondroblastoma
  Chondromucoid fibroma
  Chondrosarcoma

- Osseous—osteoma
  Osteoid osteoma
  Parosteal ossifying fibroma
  Otseogenic sarcoma
- Resorptive type
  - Bony cyst
  - Fibrous dysplasia
  - Giant cell tumor
  - Diffuse osteotitis fibrosa cystica

Type II—tumors of nonosseous origin:
- Tumours from Marro or Haversian system
  Ewing's sarcoma
  Multiple myeloma
  Xanthoma and granuloma
  Chloroma or leukemia of bone
  Histiocytoma or histiocytic lymphoma (reticular cell sarcoma)
- Metstatic
  - Carcinoma of thyroid, breast, prostate, kidneys
  - Lymphoma
  - Neuroblastoma
  - Sarcoma

Type III—by direct invasion or inclusion
  Chordoma
  Angioma
  Angiosarcoma
  Myosarcoma
  Synovioma
  Fibroma and fibrosarcoma of fascia and sheath.

Q.70 What is classification of floating knee injuries?
Ans. This is classified by Lett Wincent as follows:
- Type A—closed diaphyseal fractures
- Type B—closed metaphyseal and diaphyseal fractures
- Type C—diaphyseal fracture with epiphyseal separation
- Type D—one compound fracture with major soft tissue injury
- Type E—both compound fracture with major soft tissue injury.

Q.71 What is Enneking's classification of malignant tumours of hand?
Ans.
- Stage IA—low grade intracompartment
- Stage IB—low grade extracompartment
- Stage IIA—high grade intracompartment
- Stage IIB—high grade extracompartment
- Stage III—either grade with regional or distant metastases.

16. **W Roentgen (1845–1923)**
    Found X-rays in 1895.

17. **Willian TG Morton (1819–1868)**
    Known for anaesthesia, Morton's metatarsalgia and first laparotomy for acute appendicitis.

18. **Langenbeck (1810–1887)**
    Nailed hip fracture for the first time, known for his long instruments for non-touch technique and reducing incidence of infection.

19. **Sir William A Lane (1856–1943)**
    Used steel for instruments and implants and famous for his long handled instruments.

20. **Percival Pott (1714–1788)**
    Described Pott's Puffy tumor in the skull, Pott's paraplegia, Pott's fracture dislocation of ankle before invention of X-ray, Pott's spine and disease.

21. **Sir Benjamin Brodie (1783–1862)**
    Described Brodie's abscess and introduced fellowship examinations (1843). He was the first president of General Medical Council.

22. **WJ Little (1810–1894)**
    Described in details cerebral palsy, established tenotomy of tendo-Achilles in CTEV. He had himself left Talipes equine varus deformity.

23. **Sir James Paget (1814–1899)**
    He started as curator of Museum and Demonstrator in Anatomy and became consultant in 1847 and became President of Royal Society in 1875.

    He was not good operator but he was good orator and very good clinician and identified carpal tunnel syndrome, osteitis deformans and calcification in muscle in *Trichinella spiralis*.

24. **Madame Auguste Dejerine-Klumpke (1859–1927)**
    First lady doctor in Paris and described brachial plexus and radicular paralysis.

25. **Robert William Smith (1807–1873)**
    He described Neurofibromatosis even before Von Reck Lunghausen in 1882 and Madelung's deformity before Madelung described. He recognised Smith fracture dislocation.

26. **Ambroise Pare (1510–1590)**
    He has found method of ligation of vessels and described many surgical instruments. He is the father of French surgery and he was surgeon of Four Kings of France. He has described rupture of tendo-Achilles for the first time and described prosthesis for amputees.

27. **Richard Von Volkman (1830–1889)**
    He described Volkman's canal in bone marrow, Volkman's ligament, and Volkman's ischemic contracture of forearm. His pen name was Richard Lender.

has also published a work on "Surgical Appliances," and "Minor Operative Surgery," and in the current year he has written the article on "Diseases of the Breast".

7. **Joseph Seaton Barr (1901–1964)**

   At one time in his career, Dr Barr was extremely interested in scoliosis. In 1936, he described a three-point brace for its treatment. He was also the director of a most worthwhile survey of the treatment of scoliosis in various clinics by a Research Committee of the American Orthopedic Association. In his later, years, he published three excellent articles on the results of arthroplasty of the hip using the Moore prosthesis. One of these papers was his Robert Jones Lecture at the Royal College of Surgeons of England.

8. **Alan Graham Apley (1914–1996)**

   Alan Apley became the editor of The Journal of Bone and Joint Surgery in 1984, at the age of 70 years. It is understandable that he became a legend in his own time, and is entirely appropriate that the sixth and seventh editions have been coauthored by Louis Solomon as Apley's System of Orthopedics and Fractures.

9. **John Rhea Barton (1794–1871)**

   The literature are the paper described above, his Longitudinal Section of the Lower Jaw for the Removal of a Tumour, and his New Treatment for Certain Cases of Anchylosis.

10. **Edward Hallaran Bennett (1837–1907)**

    Bennett's first comment on fractures of the base of the first metacarpal was contained in a report to the Dublin Pathological Society in 1882.1 He published two additional papers on the subject. 2,3 At a meeting of the surgical section of the Royal Academy of Medicine in Ireland in May 1897.

11. **Roberts Jones (1857–1933)**

    Nephew of HO Thomas and founder of British Orthopaedic Association, grounded rules of tendon transfer, established orthopaedics as speciality, propagated work of HO Thomas.

12. **Arthur Sidney Blundell Bankart (1879–1951)**

    Bankart made many contributions to orthopedics, the best known being his operation for recurrent dislocation of the shoulder.

13. **Giovanni Battista Monteggia (1762–1815)**

    Started as surgical pathologist. Described fracture disloation of Monteggia of radius and ulna before the era of X-rays.

14. **BG Dupuytren (1777–1835)**

    He described contracture of hand, fractures around ankle, congenital dislocation of hip, deposits and formation of callus and subungual exostosis.

15. **John Lister**

    Lord Lister performed first operation using aseptic surgery in 1865.

CHAPTER 43

International and National Orthopaedic Surgeons Who Have Contributed to World of Orthopaedics

INTERNATIONAL

1. **Hugh Owen Thomas (1834–1891)**
   Son of bone setter known for his-Thomas' bed knee splint for lower limb and upper limb, Thomas' test of hip joint, pulled elbow, cervical collar, metatarsal bar, heel wedges

2. **Robert Adams (1791–1875)**
   In 1857, Adams published his most important contribution "A Treatise on Rheumatic Gout, or Chronic Rheumatic Arthritis of All of the Joints."

3. **Abraham Colles (1773–1843)**
   Youngest president of royal college, established role of mercury in venereal diseases, described fracture of lower end of radius with typical invered dinner fork deformity even before invention of X-rays in 1895. He walked for long distance to get his degree.

4. **David McCrae Aitken (1876–1954)**
   And as a contributor to the Robert Jones Birthday Volume of 1928 he wrote on "Curvature of the Spine." The following year he delivered his presidential address to the orthopedic Section of the Royal Society of medicine on "Respiratory Rhythm in Physiological Relation to Movement and Posture."

5. **Fred Houdlette Albee (1876–1945)**
   In 1913, Albee designed a special fracture table that became a most useful addition to the armamentarium of the orthopedic surgeon. In 1936, the table was modified by the use of a central hydraulic hoist and became known as the Albee–Comper table.
   In 1913, Albee performed his first extra-articular arthrodesis of the hip with the use of two rigid cortical grafts

6. **Thomas Annandale (1838–1971)**
   In 1864 published his Jacksonian Prize Essay on the "Malformations, Diseases, and Injuries of the Fingers and Toes, and their-388-Surgical Treatment." He

Q.72 What is Mast-Spiegel-Pappas classification of Pilon fractures?

Ans. This combines elements from previous classifications:
- *Type I*—rotational injury with vertical loading at the time of impact with malleolar fractures and fracture of posterior lip
- *Type II*—spiral extension type fracture
- *Type III*—vertical compression fracture, fracture of metaphysis and comminution of articular surface.

28. **Paul of Aegina (625–690)**
   He did first laminectomy and described ganglion for the first time.

29. **TP McMurray (1887–1949)**
   He invented his displacement osteotomy at hip for osteoarthritis of hip which was followed for fracture neck of femur also which gave good results. He wrote article on internal derangement of knee and established his test for meniscal tear of knee. He authored the *Textbook of Orthopaedics* and followed Sir Robert Jones at Liverpool.

30. **Sir William Macewen (1848–1924)**
   He devised osteotome used for osteotomy for genu valgum of rickets.

31. **Bunnel (1882–1924)**
   He known for his work on tendon transfer in hand especially in Hansen's disease hand.

32. **Surgeons Who Have Done Work On Bone Grafting**
   Jobi Meekren-1682—did first bone grafting.
   Fred Albee-1911—used cortical graft for spinal fusion (posterior)
   Phemister-1931—used cancellous bone grafts for nonunion without opening site of nonunion and laying bone grafts around it.
   Ghromley- 1933—used iliac crest bone grafts.

33. **Charnley (1911–1982)**
   Known for his excellent book on conservative methods of management of fractures in children.
      He had established Charnley's total arthroplasty of hip. He is also known for his compression arthrodesis clamps for knee and ankle arthrodesis and his operative procedure for ankle, tendo-Achilles, hip osteotomy is known very well to all.

34. **William Morrant Baker (1839–1896)**
   Known for Morrant baker cyst at knee.

35. **Walter Putnam Blount (1900–1992)**
   Blount believed strongly in nonoperative treatment and the benefits of subsequent skeletal growth and remodeling. Blount was one of the first to show the significance of old fractures as an indication of child abuse.

36. **Lorenz Böhler (1885–1973)**
   Known for his Böhler splint.

37. **David Marsh Bosworth (1897–1979)**
   Known for his Bosworth posterior fusion of spine.

38. **Harold Buhalts Boyd (1904–1981)**
   His own articles involved mainly congenital pseudarthrosis of the tibia, bone grafting for nonunion, femoral neck and trochanteric fractures, and dislocations of the shoulder. His original contributions were in the areas of dual-onlay bone grafts for nonunions, an anatomical approach for exposure of the radial head and neck and proximal end of the ulna, amputation of the

foot with tibiocalcaneal fusion, and disarticulation of the hip. He always was interested in innovations and had the ability to identify clinical applications, such as compression plates for the fixation of forearm fracture.

39. **Willis Cohoon Campbell (1880–1941)**

    He was one of the pioneers in the development of arthroplasties. He had perhaps the greatest experience in his work on arthroplasty of the knee, and he contributed extensively by his experience with the massive on lay bone graft.

ORTHOPAEDIC SURGEONS FROM INDIA WHO HAVE CONTRIBUTED TO THE WORLD OF ORTHOPAEDICS

1. **Dr BN Sinha**

    Founder President of Indian Orthopaedic Association.

2. **Dr B Mukhopadhya**

    Founder Secretary of Indian Orthopaedic Association. First Indian to deliver Hunterian lecture his work for congenital talipes equinuovarus (CTEV), Tuberculosis of bone and joint and infection is known all over world

3. **Dr PK Duraiswamy**

    First Indian to get Robert Jones medal for his experimental work on chick embryo where he had shown that by giving injection of insulin different kind of congenital deformities can be produced.

4. **Dr Katrak RJ**

    Famous for his plaster technique for CTEV. Did good work for fracture neck of femur nail and fibular graft. Known for fixation Katrak's plate for McMurray' osteotomy.

5. **Dr AK Talwalkar**

    - He designed square nails for forearm bones with principle of square peg in round hole.
    - He designed nail and plate for intertrochanteric fracture as modified Talwalkar's nail and plate like one piece
    - He also designed V nail for fracture of tibia and popularised medial entry of V nail for tibial fractures
    - He was known for doing orthopaedic operations very fast with belief that by doing fast surgery one can avoid many complications.

6. **Dr KT Dholakia**

    First Indian to become president of SICOT.
    He did first THR in India.

7. **Dr AK Gupta**

    Known for his work on Rickets and fracture neck of femur in children and founder member of Indian Orthopaedic Association.

8. **DR KS Grewal**
   Leading spine surgeon founder member of IOA and established orthopaedic surgeons in North India.

9. **Dr Balu Shankaran**
   First chairman of Artificial Limbs Manufacturing Corporation of India (ALIMCO) of India.

10. **DR M Natarajan**
    Established First Government Rehabilitation and Trauma Center in India. He described Madras Foot.

11. **Dr SM Tuli**
    Great worker for TB bone and joint, wrote Text book on this subject pioneered middle path treatment regimen for bone and joint TB.

12. **Dr PS Maini**
    - Established Singh and Maini Index of osteoporosis
    - Did lot of hip replacements, for arthritis of hip
    - Former President of IOA.

13. **Dr Varghese Chacko**
    Ex. President of IOA
    Known for his good work for Perthe's disease.

14. **Dr Min H Mehta, MD, FRCS**
    - First lady orthopaedic surgeon to get Roberts Jones Gold Medal
    - Her work for infantile scoliosis is widely accepted and appreciated (Rib Vertebral Angle).

15. **Dr PK Seth**
    - Known internationally for his Jaipur foot where person can walk bare footed and even can dance. Received Magsaysay Award-first Indian orthopaedic surgeon to get this prestigious award
    - Established rehabilitation center in Rajasthan

16. **Dr AK Shah**
    Known for his work on shoulder. Zero position and osteotomy of humerus.

17. **Dr BB Joshi**
    Internationally known as hand surgeon and for his unparallel JESS (Joshi's external stabilizing system) fixator for rigid and recurring CTEV.
    - Former president of IOA.

18. **Dr Shailendra Bhattacharya**
    Known internationally for his excellent operation for stiff elbow—Arthrolysis.

19. **Dr TK Shanmugasundaram**
    - Known for his good work of TB hip, Polio surgery
    - Established World Orthopedic Concern (WOC)
    - Ex-president of IOA

20. **Dr DP Baxi**
    - Known for his good total elbow arthroplasty-designed and developed implant for this, first orthopaedic surgeon to get NRDC award in India
    - Also known for his muscle pedicle graft
    - Former President of IOA

21. **Dr SS Yadav**
    - Known for his extensive work on fibular grafting.
    - Former President of IOA.

22. **Dr KP Daga**
    - Designed and developed first totally Indian Interlocking nail for tibial fracture where the patient are made to bear weight on the day of surgery (Daga interlocking)
    - Second orthopaedic surgeon to get NRDC award in India.

23. **Dr B Shivshanker**
    - Known for his TIC-TIC technique
    - Became president of NAILS CON

24. **Dr Sandeep Adake**
    - Started Ilizarov centre at Solapur.

25. **Dr L Prakash**
    - Inventor for knee TKR designed Indian by YTKR and good orator, and teacher and inventor of many procedures.

This is not complete list. I might have missed many more eminent orthopaedic surgeons who have made much contribution to the world of orthopaedic. Due apologies for that.

Bibliography

1. APTA Guide to Physical Therapist Practice
2. Arthritis and Allied Conditions—McCarty DJ, Koopman WJ
3. Campell's Operative Orthopaedics
4. Clinical Methods of Das
5. Clinical Methods—Dr Sureshwar Pandey
6. Computed Body Tomography with MRI Correlations—Lee JKT, Sagel SS, Stanley RJ, Heiken JP
7. Congenital Dislocation of Hip—Weinstein SL, Book of Paediatric Orthopaedics
8. Cunningham Dissection Volumes
9. Current Concepts—Dr TK Taneja
10. Diseases of Nerves of Foot—By Mann RA
11. Essentials of Nuclear Medicine Imaging—Mettler FA, Guiberteau
12. Extensile Exposure—Arnold Henry
13. Fracture Fixation—Dr AJ Thakur
14. Fractures and Joint Injuries by Sir Reginald Watson Jones
15. Hand surgery—by Edward Flynn
16. Journal of Bone and Joint Surgery—Selected volumes
17. McGregor's Surgical Anatomy
18. Modern Trends in Oprthopaedics—Vol. 3, Vol. 5
19. MRI Musculoskeletal System—Berquist TH
20. Neurological Diagnosis—Pattern
21. Nuclear Medicine in Clinical Diagnosis and Treatment —Murray
22. Oprthopaedic Surgery by Sir. Walter Mercer
23. Orthoses—Dey
24. Osteoarthritis of the hip-Bombelli R
25. OT Manual—Dr TK Taneja
26. Plaster Techniques—Kent Wu
27. Practice of Intramedullary Nailing
28. Radiology of Skeletal Trauma—Rogers LF
29. Recent Advances in Orthopaedics—A Graham Apley
30. Skeletal Tuberculosis—Prof Dr SM Tuli
31. Textbook of Anatomy—Chauarsia
32. Textbook of Orthopaedics—Rockwood Green
33. Textbook of Spinal Surgery—Bridewell KH, De-Wald RL
34. The Hip—Balderston RA
35. Traction and Splints—Stewart Hallei
36. Wheeler's Textbook of Orthopaedics